Preface

**BY RAJ DASGUPTA, M.D., ASSISTANT PROFESSOR
OF CLINICAL MEDICINE, KECK SCHOOL OF MEDICINE,
UNIVERSITY OF SOUTHERN CALIFORNIA**

As a sleep doctor and California native, I've had plenty of exposure to those who have tried substances such as CBD, THC, and everything in between. It was the firsthand experiences and countless anecdotes from my patients about the benefits of CBD that led me to take a deeper dive into understanding how it can help people. There has been a lot of red tape and limitations on the research and application of cannabis products. Nonetheless, evidence suggests that CBD may have numerous therapeutic properties and benefits in the medical world. Once we allowed ourselves to depart from the notion that cannabis is only for the "spaced-out hippies with munchies," we opened the doors to a variety of possibilities for medical application.

CBD has exploded in popularity because of its potential to treat common health problems such as pain, anxiety, and insomnia. My patients often use CBD to avoid starting new medications or as a medication alternative. I think this is great as a practitioner because now I have another tool on my belt to help my patients avoid starting medications with more high-risk side effect profiles such as narcotics, anxiolytics, and sleeping aids. It's clear that further investigation still needs to be done to determine daily dosage, route of administration, and shelf life. But what we do know now is that CBD works well for many people who have no other alternatives. It's being used all over the world, and there are countless accounts of the beneficial impact that CBD can make on an individual's life. I feel as though we are only at the early stages of understanding the therapeutic potential of this compound, and it will be exciting to see what CBD can do for humankind.

Prevention

CBD & YOU

**Straight Facts About the Plant-Based
Health Supplement for
Anxiety, Pain, Insomnia & More**

Nelson Peña & Scott Meyer
Foreword by Richard Carmona, M.D.,
17th Surgeon General of the United States

Cover design by Joanna Williams
Cover photo by Jeff Westbrook
Book design by Joanna Williams

Library of Congress Cataloging-in-Publication Data Available on Request

10 9 8 7 6 5 4 3 2 1

Published by Hearst Home, an imprint of
Hearst Books/Hearst Magazine Media, Inc.
300 West 57th Street
New York, NY 10019

Hearst Home, the Hearst Home logo, and Hearst Books are
registered trademarks of Hearst Magazine Media, Inc.
Prevention is a registered trademark of Hearst Magazines, Inc.

For information about custom editions, special sales, premium and corporate
purchases, please go to hearst.com/magazines/hearst-books

Printed in the United States of America

ISBN 978-1950785018

Contents

Foreword

BY RICHARD CARMONA, M.D.
17TH SURGEON GENERAL OF THE UNITED STATES

Like people all over the world for millennia, Americans have always sought a "magic bullet" or quick fix for what ails them. That's where enterprising sales people have eagerly stepped in, from hucksters in horse-driven wagons in the 19th century selling snake oil, to present day infomercials and social media marketers offering unregulated supplements to address all that ails you from aches to zoonoses.

We now have before us cannabidiol (CBD), a derivative of cannabis, the marijuana plant, the newest of the potential "magic bullets" that is actually a rediscovered ancient natural remedy. Certainly, our historical knowledge of numerous alleged miracle cures over the centuries would suggest that we should be very cautious of any single product that purports to be able to improve and or cure a wide range of maladies. Yet, here we are, with CBD popping up all over the country, in dozens of kinds of products, many of which make claims that rival the boldest snake oil salesmen of the past. Nonetheless, reputable researchers and others in the medical community are excited by its promise.

As with any new remedy, the story is complicated and CBD

is far from a cure-all. As surgeon general of the United States, my job description was to protect, promote, and advance the health, safety, and security of the United States. In carrying out my broad mandate, my team and I had the privilege to work with every branch of the federal government, state and local governments, NGOs, and occasionally foreign governments in order to make sure that we always had the best research and information available to ensure safety and efficacy in all our endeavors and recommendations. During my tenure, there was an ever-increasing nonscientific and anecdotally driven national movement to legalize medicinal and recreational cannabis, which included CBD. Working closely with my colleagues at the FDA, NIH, and CDC, we advised Congress and the public about the perils of such action without the appropriate scientific due diligence to ensure public safety and the appropriate utilization, if any. Although these discussions took place more than 15 years ago, our recommendations are still very relevant today.

After my tenure as the nation's surgeon general, I found that the public is more even divided, confused, and polarized regarding cannabis products, including CBD, because of the nonregulated, mostly anecdotally driven market. Claims of therapeutic value are questionable as is the purity of the product and the integrity of the supply chain.

When it comes to CBD, there is at present only one FDA approved medical use, which is the use in children with severe recurrent seizures not treatable by the usual means. The scientific examination of all things cannabis is a significantly growing field—but most information currently supporting its widespread clinical use is primarily anecdotal. This growing tsunami of anecdotal support for CBD begs for legitimate scientific research so as to clearly define its production and use from "seed to feed" while providing uniform health literate and culturally competent information to the public so that there is clearly defined "informed consent" for all CBD use.

I am proud to write this foreword in support of *Prevention* magazine and my colleagues' work. This book is an important step toward educating the public based on science and not on anecdotes or politically driven, ill-informed policy. I remain interested and open to what the future holds for CBD, provided we all take the time and effort to understand its reality.

CBD 101

THE BASICS ABOUT THE POPULAR HEALTH SUPPLEMENT EVERYONE IS TALKING ABOUT.

IN THIS CHAPTER

What Is CBD?
Your First Questions Answered
The Promise of CBD
The Concerns

As you may have heard, there's a new health supplement that's vying for a spot in your medicine cabinet. Millions of people swear by it. Others, including many doctors, aren't quite as sure, at least not yet. It's CBD, which is shorthand for cannabidiol (pronounced canna-bi-dial), a natural, plant-based chemical compound that promises to reduce anxiety, pain, insomnia, and more. And suddenly, it's everywhere.

The fact is, though much investigation into CBD is just beginning in the United States, it's been around as part of folk remedies for thousands of years. Now, as a natural compound to soothe body and mind, CBD has captured the imagination of many in the health and wellness community. "CBD is anti-inflammatory, antibacterial, antianxiety, and immunosuppressive," says Joseph Cohen, D.O., a Colorado physician. In fact, the National Academies of Sciences, Engineering, and Medicine convened a committee of experts to review cannabidiol's effect for pain and insomnia. Their report suggested positive evidence that cannabidiol could be effective. Some experts see huge potential. "The brain is about a symphony," neuroscientist Yasmin Hurd, Ph.D., told the *New York Times*, and she suspects CBD can "bring the entire symphony into harmony."

The public reaction has been even more effusive, as CBD has made a bold entry into popular culture, media, and conversations nationwide. "Everyone who buys the product comes back and raves about it—including my mother," a convenience-store clerk in North Carolina told the *Washington Post*. Elsewhere, one fan said, "Physically, it's like taking a warm bath, melting the tension away." When *Prevention* asked readers to share their CBD experiences, many responded with positive stories. "I use it twice a day," one accountant wrote. "I also take it for pain and have been able to drastically reduce the amount of Advil and Aleve that I was taking on a daily basis."

This book will provide just enough science and history to help you understand cannabidiol, but more important, it contains useful advice about considering, buying, and using CBD. Inside, you'll find a condition-by-condition guide based on the most credible research available (starting on page 89), an objective discussion of the hype around CBD (page 30), as well as some of the limitations, unknowns, doubts, and serious questions to consider, along with insight on CBD's intriguing potential (page 20).

WHAT IS CBD?

CBD is one of more than 100 compounds known as cannabinoids, which are found in cannabis plants. Yes, CBD is from cannabis, but there are many different strains of the cannabis plant. Some strains are high in the chemical compound tetrahydro-cannabinol (THC). Legally, in the United States, any cannabis strain with more than 0.3 percent THC is considered marijuana, famous for its psychoactive effects. There are other strains that contain high concentrations of CBD with little or no THC. Strains of cannabis with less than 0.3 percent of THC are known as hemp. CBD extracted from hemp plants does not have psychoactive effects, and it is this compound that's found in the products available to you.

CBD doesn't get you high, but according to proponents, it can bring relief to the body and mind in important ways, which is why it's become a wellness phenomenon. In fact, these days, it's more talked about than its well-known psychoactive sibling, THC. On Google, CBD passed THC in 2016 as the most widely searched cannabis compound. Today, it's not even close. There are now more than three times as many searches for CBD every month. A 2019 Harris Poll found that 86 percent of US adults had heard of CBD and 18 percent had tried it—an impressive profile for a plant extract that was almost completely unknown just a few years ago.

The main reason for cannabidiol's explosive growth? Early adopters—the people using CBD right now to help them with anxiety, insomnia, pain, or other conditions—often say that it's effective. In a 2019 *Prevention* survey, more than two-thirds of CBD users said that it worked as they had hoped. In fact, 81 percent said they would be willing to spend $30 to $50 a month for cannabidiol. (Almost one in five said they'd pay at least $100 a month to keep their medicine cabinet stocked with CBD.) Overall, 78 percent said they'd recommend it.

This doesn't mean the appeal is universal. In the *Prevention* survey, more than 20 percent said it didn't work for them as they had hoped. But the experiences of the majority are creating a rare grassroots movement—a health-product boom that did not begin from big pharmaceutical companies. This compound, with its unique and fascinating history, is changing the landscape of how millions of Americans approach their health and wellness.

Of course, big business has noticed. When New York–based investment bank Cowen & Company studied the booming CBD market in 2018, they found that it was already between a $600 million and $2 billion business in the United States. (For comparison, the entire noncannabis herbal supplement market in 2017 was estimated at about $1 billion.) Even more striking: Cowen estimates that by 2025, the cannabidiol market will be $16 billion. The CBD research and analytics firm Brightfield Group is even more bullish, predicting that the

CBD market will pass $23 billion by 2023, which would almost match the current revenue of Starbucks. "There is too much momentum . . . for this industry not to explode," the group wrote. "Setting about sizing this market led us to speak with hundreds of people and crunch tens of thousands of numbers, leading us to understand that the hemp-derived CBD market is indeed growing at a breathtaking pace."

66 My Take

I have pain in my lower back, shin splints in my left leg, and sciatica that affects my back and legs. I purchased a jar of CBD cream for $59. The salesperson said it would take about two weeks to be effective. I also purchased at the same time dark chocolate infused with CBD for about $22. They were somewhat effective together the first three days. But, when the chocolate ran out, not so much. I next bought a tincture. It was 500 milligrams for $49. It worked much better with the cream. I still could feel some pain, but at a lesser intensity. On my third week I bought an accelerant cream with 2,400 milligrams of CBD in the 2.5-ounce container. It was $79. It appears to help a little better. But the pain is still there. Overall, CBD is not as effective for me at the prices presently required for its purchase. **—LaVerne Saunders, Chicago, Illinois**

Where that growth will lead is hard to predict. But this is clear: CBD has captured the attention of the general public, and its popularity is soaring. There are countless companies selling CBD online, and it only takes a visit to a convenience store, health food store, drug store, supermarket, gas station—

or that new CBD store that just popped up down the street—
to find cannabidiol for sale near you, in a wide variety of forms.
CBD can be purchased in oils, drops, creams, capsules, gummies, soaps, toothpicks, beard oil, breath sprays, lip balm, bath
salts, pet products, and more. Seven percent of American
adults use CBD, according to 2019 consumer surveys by both
Harris and Cowen & Company. This translates to nearly
18 million US adults—and growing.

> **Remember This:** To help with anxiety, pain, inflammation,
> and insomnia, lots of people are using CBD, a natural,
> nonpsychoactive compound found in high concentration in
> hemp, a strain of cannabis.

YOUR FIRST QUESTIONS ANSWERED

Cannabidiol's newfound popularity raises some compelling
questions, such as the following:

HOW COME I NEVER HEARD OF IT UNTIL RECENTLY?

Call it guilt by association. CBD isn't truly new, but for almost
80 years it was largely hidden from the public because it
comes from the cannabis plant. Until recent years, cannabis
was illegal in all US states. Decades ago when authorities
began cracking down on marijuana, the research and distri-
bution of CBD in the United States stopped almost completely. (For more on the fascinating history of CBD, see
Chapter 2.)

HOW DOES CBD WORK IN THE BODY?

Your body contains the endocannabinoid system, a network of receptors featuring key molecules known as cannabinoids. This network acts as a signaling system. When faced with a challenge, your body's natural cannabinoids alert your system that hormones and other responses are needed to keep things in balance. For instance, if you overheat, this system alerts your body to sweat. You don't store these internal cannabinoids in your body—you produce them only when they're needed.

But here's where it gets interesting. Remarkably, the cannabis plant produces cannabinoids as well. These were first discovered back in the 1940s, but were not as well understood until the 1990s. Scientists ultimately found that, when ingested, some of the plant's cannabinoid compounds act similarly to the cannabinoids our bodies produce. One of the most compelling of these is cannabidiol, or CBD. According to CBD advocates, by ingesting CBD, you can complement your natural supply of cannabinoids and better arm your body to respond to challenges such as stress.

WHAT BENEFITS DOES IT BRING?

Because of the long ban on research in the United States, most of the studies on CBD are recent, short-term, and conducted on animals, not humans. But, to many observers, the research is encouraging. Studies involving rats and mice have shown that CBD has positive effects for pain, inflammation, and anxiety. And early research on humans shows promise for CBD as a sleep aid.

Meanwhile, anecdotal evidence is piling up, as millions of people try CBD and report their results to friends, doctors, and online. (Sprinkled throughout this book, you will find a sampling of these stories under the heading "My Take.") Some people are disappointed and say the results are less than they expected, especially for the relatively high cost. (Prices vary, but a 30-count bottle of 25 milligram capsules often costs $60 or more.) But for others, it's a small price to pay for what they say is true relief. Many report benefits for pain, anxiety, headache, insomnia, and other issues, including symptoms related to inflammation, menopause, and menstruation. Supporters often tout the advantage of taking a natural product with few if any side effects or risk of addiction, rather than relying on pharmaceutical medications, including opioids.

IS IT LEGAL?

Unlike marijuana, which is legal in some states, illegal in others, and still frowned upon by federal authorities, hemp—and the CBD that comes from it—is generally considered legal to possess and use according to the US federal government. This is the result of the Farm Bill passed by Congress in 2018 (The law is new enough that legal interpretations are still subject to change. Check before buying.). In states that have legalized marijuana, it is legal to produce and sell CBD harvested from the marijuana plant. Elsewhere, CBD products come from hemp and are generally legal and available with no prescription required.

There are some exceptions. Two states—Nebraska and South Dakota—have yet to catch up with the federal law, and

CBD products are still illegal there. In addition, Idaho follows stricter regulations than the federal law, effectively making many CBD products illegal there. In late 2019, the US Food and Drug Administration (FDA) released a statement declaring that it is illegal to market CBD as a food additive or dietary supplement, noting that it would continue to review the science and update its regulations as needed. (For more on CBD's legal status, see page 56.)

IS IT RISKY?

CBD is generally considered safe, though the FDA noted in 2019 that the safety data is based on limited science and unanswered questions remain. With all the new usage of cannabidiol, there have been some minor side effects reported (see page 76), but for many people, there are no unexpected impacts at all. The good news so far: In most human studies involving CBD, only a small percentage of users have difficulty tolerating it. Cannabidiol is also known to be nonaddictive. Many doctors remain unsure whether CBD is effective or an example of the placebo effect— but even skeptics in the medical community generally consider it rather harmless (unless a patient with a serious illness uses it to replace a more proven medical treatment). Another major caution: The CBD that's available in shops or online is currently subject to no government regulation, which means it may contain other ingredients or not even be CBD at all. It's often advised that buyers research cannabidiol companies to make sure they are reputable, look for product lab reports and ingredient lists on websites, read reviews, and start with small doses. (For much more on buying smart, see Chapter 5.)

THE PROMISE OF CBD

Someday, science may have a full handle on exactly what CBD can and cannot do. But that day has yet to come. In the absence of long-term, double-blind, randomized, placebo-controlled human studies on cannabidiol's effects, some proponents (with perhaps some wishful thinking) have created a long and inclusive list of potential powers for this little plant extract. The possibilities sometimes touted include help for acne, addiction, Alzheimer's, anorexia, appetite reduction, beauty, cancer, depression, diabetes, digestive issues, glaucoma, heart disease, menstrual relief, migraines, multiple sclerosis, muscle spasms, nausea, nerve issues, Parkinson's, post-traumatic stress disorder (PTSD), schizophrenia, sexual enhancement, skin care, weight loss, and more.

For some of these issues, no CBD-related relief may ever come. But for some others, researchers are already encouraged. One example is Esther Blessing, Ph.D., an assistant professor at New York University's School of Medicine, whose research investigates CBD as a treatment for PTSD and alcohol use disorder. "CBD is the most promising drug that has come out for neuropsychiatric diseases in the last 50 years," Blessing told the *New York Times* in 2018. "The reason it is so promising is that it has a unique combination of safety and effectiveness over a very broad range of conditions."

Other research is showing that CBD may, at some point, play a role in quelling the deadly opioid epidemic. A 2015 study published in the journal *Neurotherapeutics* indicated that non-habit-forming CBD might help recovering opioid addicts avoid relapse, likely by reducing anxiety and cravings.

For most serious conditions, much more research is needed. As far back as 2012, a review of studies published in the *British Journal of Clinical Pharmacology* reported the far-from-definitive but nonetheless intriguing news that "evidence is emerging to suggest that CBD is a potent inhibitor of both cancer growth and spread." Since then, research has not confirmed this early speculation, but more study is underway. A 2017 report from the National Academies of Sciences, Engineering, and Medicine found substantial evidence that cannabis (including both THC and CBD) is effective in treating muscle spasms and stiffness due to multiple sclerosis and helps with nausea and vomiting after chemotherapy. In an often-quoted Spanish study from 2010, an oral spray that included CBD was shown in a clinical trial to ward off those same chemotherapy effects.

Even when such hopeful signs emerge, medical experts caution that these are individual studies that, on their own, reveal only a small piece of the puzzle. More work is needed to understand CBD's full value and limitations. (For a condition-by-condition listing, see Chapter 4.)

MOST POPULAR USES

While all kinds of future purposes for CBD may still be unrecognized or under early investigation, there are millions of people using it right now for anxiety, sleeplessness, inflammation, and pain. As CBD makes its splashy debut on the consciousness of health-minded people everywhere, it is being used for many conditions, but at its core, the public appeal so far centers on this tight circle of concerns. Most users don't take it for general health and well-being, but rather to bring relief for a specific problem. In the 2019 *Prevention* CBD survey, people who had used CBD were asked to share their reasons (as many as they liked) and were given a variety of options to choose from. Of more than 800 total responses, 56 percent cited pain, while 48 percent said it was for anxiety; 32 percent included inflammation, and one in four chose insomnia. It's a reality that plays out wherever CBD proponents gather. Online and in retail shops, the consistency is striking.

A 2019 Harris Poll found similar results. For this survey, while inflammation wasn't offered as a choice, the other top responses struck a familiar chord. Fifty-five percent said they used CBD for relaxation, while 50 percent chose stress and anxiety relief. Forty-five percent cited sleep, while 44 percent said it was to treat muscle pain. (Other types of pains also scored high.) Scan the comment section for any online CBD product and you'll note the same trend.

Stress and Sleep

It's not surprising that a cannabis extract may be relaxing and sleep-inducing. After all, marijuana enthusiasts have been noticing the same effect for generations. In fact, part of that reaction has always been due to CBD, which is a natural compound in marijuana as well as in hemp. While CBD lacks the psychoactive power of THC, experts say it still can transform your mood. "CBD does change cognition," says Jahan Marcu, Ph.D., COO, and director of experimental pharmacology and behavioral research at the International Research Center on Cannabis and Mental Health, in New York City. "CBD goes into the brain, where it affects receptors associated with mood, which is why people take it for anxiety." With less anxiety often comes better sleep. Even a rare study from the 1980s showed that subjects who took 160 milligrams of CBD slept longer than those who took a placebo.

In 2018, Scott Shannon, M.D., assistant clinical professor at the University of Colorado, examined the records of 72 patients who used CBD for three months to help with anxiety and sleep. In the resulting study, which was published in the *Permanente Journal*, Dr. Shannon found "a fairly rapid decrease in anxiety scores that appears to persist for months." In fact, anxiety scores decreased within the first month in 57 of the 72 patients and remained low. Dr. Shannon notes that at a time of great CBD hype, it is possible the placebo effect may have played a role, but he concludes that while more research is certainly needed, "cannabidiol may hold benefit for anxiety-related disorders."

Research results do vary. In a double-blind human study at the University of Chicago, subjects were given CBD and then shown unpleasant images or words. The idea was to see if the calming effects of cannabidiol could help them handle the negative stimuli better than a control group. But, in this study, there was no difference in the emotional reaction of the CBD and placebo groups.

More intense: A 2012 study published in the journal *Neuro-psychopharmacology*, in which Brazilian scientists pretreated mice with CBD and had them chased by a snake through a maze—clearly an anxiety-invoking situation. The CBD-fueled mice showed fewer panicked responses than those that received the placebo, and researchers concluded that they experienced less panic and fear. Even better news: All the mice survived this harrowing experience. And the point was made: Even in the toughest situations, at least according to this study, CBD can indeed be helpful with anxiety.

Pain and Inflammation

A majority of CBD users cited chronic pain and arthritis pain as their main reasons for trying CBD, according to a paper published in the journal *Cannabis and Cannabinoid Research*. It's understandable. The CBD-pain connection has been long noted and remains persistent in the research. In a 2012 study using rodents, the National Institutes of Health found that "cannabinoids significantly suppress chronic inflammatory and neuropathic pain . . . (and) may represent a novel class of therapeutic agents for the treatment of chronic pain." Since then, some other research has confirmed the optimism. A 2016 study using rodents published in the *European Journal of Pain* concluded that "topical CBD application has therapeutic potential for relief of arthritis pain-related behaviors and inflammation without evident side-effects."

Some experts say that for CBD to be truly effective, it needs to be paired with THC, as it is in medical marijuana. There's a fairly broad consensus for the effectiveness of medical marijuana as a pain reliever. That 2017 report from the National Academies of Sciences, Engineering, and Medicine said there was "conclusive or substantial evidence" that cannabis (including THC and CBD) is effective in treating chronic pain. A year later, Serbian scientists reviewed studies on medical cannabis (again, including both THC and CBD) and concluded that "the evidence from current research supports the use of medical cannabis in the treatment of chronic pain in adults."

The question is how effective is CBD on its own. The full answer will require much further research, but proponents see reasons for optimism. For instance, an article by Thorston Rudroff, Ph.D and Jacob Sosnoff, Ph.D. in *Frontiers in Neurology* said that CBD can reduce inflammation in the body and help improve pain and mobility in patients with multiple sclerosis. "It is anti-inflammatory, antioxidative, antiemetic, antipsychotic and neuroprotective," the review study authors wrote. Translation: As an antioxidant, CBD removes potentially damaging agents from the body. As an antiemetic, it is believed to be helpful in reducing nausea and vomiting. As an antipsychotic, it's thought to be potentially effective against psychosis. As a neuroprotective, it may shield nerve cells from damage.

But it's CBD's promise as an anti-inflammatory that may be most exciting of all. If it can be proven to curb inflammation throughout the body, CBD would have enormous potential as a pain reliever and more. In a 2012 review, a researcher at the University of Mississippi found that CBD works as an anti-inflammatory in the tradition of popular drugstore over-the-counter pain medications (think Tylenol, Advil, Motrin). In fact, some observers have noted similarities between CBD and aspirin. For example, both come from a plant—in the case of aspirin, the active ingredient, salicylate, was first extracted from willow bark. Like CBD, aspirin had a long history as a popular natural healing remedy for centuries before taking its place in virtually every medicine cabinet in America.

For CBD, the potential may be even bigger than that—or not—but science will tell. A wide range of chronic disorders can be traced back to inflammation and oxidative stress (which is a potentially damaging imbalance between free radicals and antioxidants in your body). This can play a key role in conditions including schizophrenia, multiple sclerosis, rheumatoid arthritis, metabolic disorders, Alzheimer's disease, Parkinson's disease, diabetes, heart disease, short-term infections, and other ailments. The 2018 Serbian study noted that "inflammation and oxidative stress are intimately involved in the genesis of many human diseases," concluding on a hopeful note that "the therapeutic utility of CBD is a relatively new area of investigation that portends new discoveries on the interplay between inflammation and oxidative stress, a relationship that underlies tissue and organ damage in many human diseases."

When it comes to pain and inflammation, CBD's biggest fans aren't waiting for the scientists to catch up. They're trying it and often reporting relief. What's more, a large number are sharing the benefits with their friends—including their pets. Almost 40 percent of dog owners (and a third of cat owners) like the idea of CBD supplements for their pets, according to research by the marketing research firm Packaged Facts. There may be some reason for their optimism. A 2019 study at Cornell University College of Veterinary Medicine found that when dogs with arthritic joint pain were treated with CBD rather than a placebo, they showed a significant decrease in pain and increase in activity, with no discernible side effects.

> **Remember This:** While early research shows potential for CBD, the studies have been relatively short term and usually not done on humans. There's much still to learn.

SEAL OF APPROVAL

While cannabidiol is being studied for all kinds of diseases and being used for familiar everyday concerns like relieving pain and sleeping better, it's only been officially approved by the FDA for two particularly brutal childhood epilepsy syndromes known as Dravet syndrome and Lennox-Gastaut syndrome.

These conditions typically don't respond to antiseizure medications. In multiple studies, extremely high doses of CBD reduced the number of seizures significantly and in some cases were able to stop the seizures altogether. In a field that normally sticks to the driest of language, the unbridled excitement of one 2017 Italian study is telling: "These are exciting times for research in cannabinoids," wrote a researcher. "After almost four millennia of their documented medical use in the treatment of seizure disorders, we are very close to obtaining conclusive evidence of their efficacy in some severe epilepsy syndromes. The era of evidence-based prescription of a cannabis product is within our sight." The researcher, Emilio Perucca, was right. In 2018, the FDA approved a drug called Epidiolex specifically for these severe conditions.

Unlike drugs that synthetically mimic parts of the cannabis

plant, Epidiolex is all natural, coming completely from the cannabis plant and containing only CBD. It's not yet certain exactly how Epidiolex works. It may inhibit or slow down the way signals are sent to the brain. Some researchers think Epidiolex adjusts how much calcium can get inside the nerves. When a nerve cell has too much calcium, it fires electric pulses too fast. These electrical overloads cause damage inside the cell during seizures. The CBD medication appears to maintain a healthy balance of calcium in those nerve cells. Like most medications, it doesn't work for everyone, but clinical trials found that seizures decreased, on average by about half.

It worked even better than that for Billy Caldwell, an 11-year-old boy in Northern Ireland who in 2017 became the first person to receive a prescription for medical cannabis in the UK. He had been suffering as many as 100 seizures per day, according to his mother, Charlotte Caldwell. These seizures amounted to a beating on his brain that seemed destined to lead to his death. But that destiny changed when in the first 300 days after his CBD prescription, Billy suffered zero seizures. (By the summer of 2019, Northern Irish authorities had reversed course and blocked doctors from prescribing medical cannabis, forcing the Caldwells into a legal challenge to keep receiving the product legally.)

From the start, the story of CBD and epilepsy is the tale of parents fighting (and innovating) to save their children. Neuro-scientist Catherine Jacobson, Ph.D., took up the battle when her own son was suffering seizures as a baby. Using her insights as a researcher, Jacobson became a central figure in CBD's incredibly fast rise in the epilepsy community. As more parents of suffering children discovered the potential of CBD, the pressure mounted on officials to speed through trials, to make it more widely available, and to legalize it. In a field where drug development and approvals can be interminably long and tedious, parents helped CBD to go from obscurity to full FDA approval in a remarkable six years.

The story was so powerful it was featured in a memorable 2019 *New York Times Magazine* article, authored by Moises Velasquez-Manoff, who wrote: "Epidiolex is also noteworthy for its unusual history. Drugs are typically developed in the lab and go through trials before reaching patients. But in the case of Epidiolex, two mothers of epileptic children experimented on their own sons and then helped push a version of what they discovered into the FDA pipeline. 'In the modern era, it's certainly the most striking example of a drug that has gone from patient use to drug development,' Ken Mackie, a neuroscientist at Indiana University, told me. And it's unlikely to be the last such example. Because so many people already use cannabis and think it helps, patients might be, in effect, pioneering new uses through self-experimentation."

In other words, medical science still doesn't exactly know everything CBD can do. Some of those answers may ultimately be discovered by the people who are using CBD now. As the epilepsy story shows, CBD has developed as a kind of folk movement, popular among the people long before governments know enough to approve. And that trend continues today.

It's no surprise that some of the medical community has

taken its usual and understandable approach: caution. Perhaps the surprise is how quickly everyday people have come to love CBD. In the 2019 *Prevention* survey, 72 percent of users rated their experience with CBD as good or very good. Only 3 percent said it was bad or very bad. Other polls show similar results. In the 2018 survey in the journal *Cannabis and Cannabinoid Research*, large percentages reported success with CBD, with 35 percent giving it the highest grade. Only 4 percent said it didn't work for them at all. In a 2019 Gallup poll of those familiar with CBD, 78 percent said it had at least some health benefits and a sizable portion (a third overall) said cannabidiol delivered a lot of health benefits. Only 4 percent said it didn't have any. More than six in ten respondents favored its availability over the counter, while only 4 percent believed it shouldn't be for sale at all—a surprising acceptance for an extract that comes from a plant as historically controversial as cannabis.

> **Remember This:** It's unclear how much CBD can ultimately help various conditions, but it's already gained millions of fans who believe in its efficacy and also has been approved by the FDA for epilepsy sufferers, bringing many of them tremendous relief.

THE CONCERNS

CBD has gained popularity so fast that many people are suspicious—that it's just a fad, that it's an example of the placebo effect, that it's not based on real science. Some worry that it's not been vetted enough to be truly safe, or that—since it's largely unregulated—it's impossible to know what you're getting when you buy it. These are legitimate concerns worth exploring.

One informed skeptic is Pal Pacher, M.D., Ph.D., an investigator at the National Institutes of Health and former president of the International Cannabinoid Research Society. After many years of studying the issue, Dr. Pacher says that there's no real proof that CBD works as well as proponents say, except in the case of epilepsy. He stresses that more research is needed.

"There are numerous animal studies which show different benefits, but none of these were confirmed in clinical studies so far, and several were actually shown in clinical trials to fail," Dr. Pacher says. "It is relatively safe, so I have no problem if people want to take it. And if they feel better, that's fine. As far as we know, though, this may all be mostly a placebo effect. The placebo effect is very, very strong."

As a respected researcher on the topic, Dr. Pacher set off alarm bells in the CBD world when he was quoted in *Newsweek* saying that the CBD phenomenon amounts to "one of the largest uncontrolled clinical trials in history, and no one really knows what it is they're taking. Everybody is being sucked into the big hype." He worries that, without solid, long-term research, CBD's buzz is way ahead of the science. To some degree, the FDA agrees. "There are many unanswered questions about the science, safety, and quality of products containing CBD," the FDA wrote in a 2019 consumer update.

Even the most ardent CBD proponents would concede a relative lack of rigorous human-based studies that are scientifically rock solid (meaning long-term, double-blind, and placebo-controlled), illustrating the benefits of cannabidiol in a virtually unassailable way. Those same proponents might also point out that there also hasn't been a torrent of such research showing that CBD doesn't work either. Both points are true. Some of the most talked-about research has come from observational studies, which follow patients' improvement after taking CBD, without the scientific controls that would make the research more valid. The only exception is in the study of seizures. In the run-up to FDA approval for Epidiolex, promising human-based studies were completed, though there hasn't been enough time yet for long-term research. For other uses, the formal study of CBD is still in its infancy.

Not all experts are as skeptical as Dr. Pacher, but all agree more study is needed. "The basic science and preclinical research is quite strong," says Dr. Shannon, the Colorado psychiatrist who has studied the effects of CBD on sleep and anxiety. "We have a good understanding of why this is likely to be a useful medical intervention. But we have little good data in humans."

ON DOUBT AND DOSAGE

Some studies that have gained positive attention for CBD are often much smaller than what is expected when investigating a new treatment or drug. A 2011 Brazilian study is often cited by CBD advocates for showing that cannabidiol lowered anxiety and discomfort for people involved in a public-speaking exercise. What got less attention: The study involved just two dozen people. Other studies are even smaller.

For some researchers, small or short-term studies are too flimsy for solid conclusions. The evidence is too scant for Frederico Garcia, M.D., Ph.D., a professor at Brazil's Federal University of Minas Gerais. In 2017, he looked at the CBD-related research for psychiatric conditions for an article published in the *World Journal of Biological Psychiatry* and concluded that he couldn't recommend it, despite the fact that many of his colleagues were excited by cannabidiol's potential. "CBD is being touted as safe and effective for several psychiatric disorders, but the data available do not prove that. The results of our review demonstrate that the use of CBD for psychiatric disorders should be regarded with caution." Such disagreements among medical experts are now common.

The fact is, trial and error doesn't happen instantly, and progress isn't always a straight line. Even some of the studies commonly cited by CBD supporters show uneven results. The Colorado anxiety report cited earlier in this chapter (page 23), for instance, also looked at the effect of CBD on sleep. For anxiety, nearly 80 percent of CBD users saw improvement that persisted for the three-month study, a fact that garnered headlines and mentions in various media. For sleep, it was a different story. Two-thirds of patients did see improvement in their sleep in the first month, but those benefits soon faded. This fact got considerably less attention. Does it mean the brain builds up a tolerance? Perhaps time will tell. Meanwhile, other studies have found the exact opposite, with CBD providing impressive benefits for sleep but not anxiety.

Such mixed results are not unusual—for CBD or anything else. Even a proven pain reliever like Tylenol fails in some trials. And doctors often caution that no substance works for each person's body in the same way. With CBD, some users report relief. Others feel nothing. With all the attention on cannabidiol, study results are interpreted and applied in real time, as they happen. In some cases, if the result isn't stellar, it's seen as a failure for CBD, when in fact, it may be exactly that, or maybe it was just the wrong dose.

Since much remains unknown about CBD, there are many questions about the right amount necessary for various uses. One piece of common dosing advice is to start with 10 milligrams and adjust upward. More aggressive guidance recommends taking 1 to 6 milligrams for every 10 pounds of body weight, then adjust within that wide range depending on results. But unlike most medications, no one knows the perfect dose.

The majority of medical professionals—especially the ones who work with patients every day—have virtually no training in the area of cannabidiol, which means they can't help much on questions such as dosage. Their medical-school textbooks surely didn't focus on obscure old folk remedies from the cannabis plant. (The good news: Professional seminars about CBD are suddenly popular as doctors scramble to understand how it works and what to advise.)

Dr. Pacher, the leading cannabidiol NIH researcher who has reviewed virtually every CBD study, notes that the rodents in the studies are almost always very small, yet the dose of CBD remains relatively large. "In most of the studies, CBD was effective for the rodents at around 10 milligrams per kilogram of body weight," Dr. Pacher says. This translates to 10 milligrams for every 2.2 pounds. "This means in a person of 80 kilograms [about 175 pounds] you might need a single dose of 800 milligrams."

Dr. Pacher's point is that most people are getting a whole lot less than that. "When you buy a cannabidiol product, usually it contains 100 to 500 milligrams in a whole vial, which you might be taking for a month or something like that. It would mean the dose that you are consuming is ten- to one hundredfold less than any dose that has been proven in any animal or human trial."

Researchers are currently experimenting with different amounts in their studies. In the long term, this will yield insights that will help users zero in on exactly how much CBD they need. These are measures that science works out through years of study. After all, there was a time when experts were still tweaking how many aspirin a patient might require for relief. It took time and research to figure it out. This is currently just beginning to happen for cannabidiol. But, of course, in the hyped CBD environment, many people are diving in and trying to figure it out for themselves.

In that Brazilian public-speaking study, subjects lowered their anxicty when treated with a megadose of 600 milligrams of CBD—that's higher than an entire typical 500-milligram bottle of tincture and much more than almost all CBD users ever take at one time. A different 2017 study gave varying doses of CBD to 60 volunteers for a single public-speaking test. It found that those who took 300 milligrams showed lower anxiety than those who took 100 milligrams or 900 milligrams. What's a potential CBD buyer to think? (For a general dosage recommendation, turn to page 89.)

66 My Take

My experience with CBD oil is that it does relieve arthritic pain in large joints (hips, knees, shoulders), as well as the neck, wrists, and thumb joint. It is also effective for helping me to fall asleep at night. I take 25 milligrams twice a day: noon and bedtime. If I wake up in pain during the night, I take another dose (5 to 6 hours after the bedtime dose), which relieves the pain and helps me get back to sleep. It does cause "dry mouth," but only when I take it during the night when I am in bed.

But all CBD oil isn't created equal. Some brands are inferior to others. It's best to buy a name brand that has a good reputation. Advil, Aleve, Ibuprofen did not work for me, which is probably good as long-term use of these products can cause intestinal bleeding and other problems. For me, CBD has no such side effects.

—C. W., Seattle, Washington

99

QUALITY CONTROL

While most experts consider CBD to be safe, and many are confident that further research will confirm some level of effectiveness, there remains a major concern when it comes to the CBD that you can purchase. In this new, unregulated field, it's hard to be completely sure that what you buy is what you think it is. There's no regulation, which means unscrupulous or sloppy manufacturers can bottle whatever they like under the name CBD.

"This market is largely buyer beware—with unlicensed manufacturers and sellers promoting a non-standardized product," says Paul Armentano, deputy director of the National Organization for the Reform of Marijuana Laws (NORML). Terms like "snake oil," "free-for-all," and "wild West" often pop up when medical experts are discussing CBD, and the fact is that some CBD is mislabeled or contaminated or contains dangerous ingredients. When Virginia Commonwealth University researchers chemically analyzed nine CBD vaping liquids, they discovered that four of the nine contained the dangerous synthetic cannabinoid known as Spice, and one had the cough suppressant dextromethorphan. In a 2017 study in the *Journal of the American Medical Association (JAMA),* the amount of CBD for most of the products tested didn't match the label. At the time, one of the study's coauthors said "there's a 75 percent chance of getting a product where the CBD is mislabeled."

This isn't just an American problem. When Britain's Centre for Medicinal Cannabis bought CBD oil for testing, it found that more than half of the purchased products did not contain the level of CBD promised on the label. Dr. Pacher describes a report presented at a recent meeting of the International Cannabis Research Society. "The researchers got CBD from approved vendors. It was quite shocking," he says. "In some of the products there was no CBD. In other products, there was

CBD but it was heavily contaminated with THC. So, let's say it's effective. You will never know what is really causing the effect. How will you reproduce it? Maybe next time you will get something different. That's the problem. You don't really know what you're taking."

The worries have clearly filtered down to the buying public. In the 2019 *Prevention* survey, when respondents were asked about their biggest CBD concerns, the two most commonly chosen responses were "I can't be sure of the quality" (46 percent) and "not sure if it's safe" (28 percent).

State governments and the CBD industry recognize the problem and are stepping in to try to bring some standardization to the field. Colorado and Oregon have laws to ensure that CBD isn't tainted by too much THC or by other contaminants. Indiana and Utah require CBD products that are sold at retail stores to include a QR code, which allows consumers to instantly check out the product's "certificate of analysis" (COA), showing the testing the company did and the exact levels of CBD and THC. An industry group called the US Hemp Authority (ushempauthority.org) provides certified seals to companies that meet specific quality standards. (For a complete guide to buying CBD smartly and safely, see Chapter 5.)

> **Remember This:** The benefits of CBD have yet to be verified by years of solid study, and product quality control and proper dosing strategies aren't yet standardized.

THE RISE OF CBD

A BRIEF LOOK AT THE INCREDIBLE HISTORY OF CBD AND THE CURRENT BOOM.

IN THIS CHAPTER

American Grown
Prohibition
Breakthroughs
The Boom
Legal Confusion, Then Clarity

While the current CBD phenomenon has put hemp in the spotlight, this versatile strain of cannabis is no newcomer. In fact, experts believe it was one of the first crops grown when humans first developed the idea of agriculture, more than 10,000 years ago. In Taiwan, scientists have found evidence of hemp cultivation in an early civilization that existed there as long as 12,000 years ago. Archaeologists have discovered ancient Chinese pottery that includes impressions from hemp rope. In those centuries as civilizations and agriculture grew, resourceful growers used hemp for cloth, rope, food, and when the cannabis strain leaned toward more THC, intoxication.

Cultures around the world recognized the healing properties of the cannabis plant early on. While most of the ancient texts don't distinguish between marijuana and hemp, it's often assumed that the medicinal properties written about were marijuana, which includes CBD and THC. An early medical use, perhaps the first, has been traced back to China in about 2,900 BC, with cannabis being used to ease menstruation and joint pain. In fact, in traditional Chinese medicine, cannabis is on the list as one of the "50 fundamental herbs." In India, ancient writings recognized the psychoactive element of cannabis, and it was used to treat headaches, insomnia, gastrointestinal disorders, and the pain of childbirth. The Ebers Papyrus, an ancient Egyptian medical textbook, mentions the use of cannabis to help with pain relief, depression, eye issues, and even hemorrhoids. (Cannabis was also used for spiritual reasons, and traces have been found on numerous mummies from ancient times, including the Pharaoh Ramesses II.)

In Russia, hemp was an ingredient in early folk remedies to treat toothaches and was used for centuries in a variety of ways, later becoming a major export. When droughts hit, the Russian poor relied on hemp seed oil for nutrition.

The *Materia Medica*—the widely influential guide to herbal medicine written in the first century by a Greek physician and botanist—describes how cannabis could help with earaches and inflammation (and, interestingly, decreasing sexual desire). The book was widely read and followed for more than 1,500 years by a variety of Western cultures.

All the while, hemp was also serving many industrial uses. When shipbuilding gained popularity, there was suddenly a major need for strong sails, lines, and ropes. Hemp filled this need. In 1588, when the English fleet defeated the Spanish Armada, British ships were carrying more than 10,000 acres of cultivated hemp, according to an estimate by historian Martin Booth. As the British Navy became a critical part of England's military power, hemp became so important that English farmers were required to grow it among their crops, risking a substantial fine if they didn't comply. By 1632, that requirement was extended to the colonies that were just developing in the Americas. The Virginia Assembly decreed "that every planter as soone as he may, provide seede of flaxe and hempe and sowe the same." Massachusetts and Connecticut had similar laws. For these early American farmers, it was illegal to *not* grow hemp.

> **Remember This:** CBD may seem like a new phenomenon, but the plants it comes from have been used for healing for thousands of years.

AMERICAN GROWN

On the ships that brought colonists to America, the sails were made of hemp. Early American currency included the image of hemp. George Washington grew it (though in one journal entry he lamented that his crop was likely to go bad because he "began to separate the male from the female hemp, rather too late."). In colonial times, hemp was made into clothing and rope and its strong fibers were used for industrial purposes. Thomas Jefferson wrote that hemp "is abundantly productive and will grow for ever on the same spot," unlike tobacco, which depletes soil nutrients. In 1763, John Adams, in a satirical letter to the *Boston Evening Post,* using the pseudonym Humphrey Plough-jogger, wrote extensively about hemp. "I do say it would be a nice thing if we could raise enuff Hemp to pay our rates, and bye a little rum and shuger, which we cant well do without ..." Adams wrote. He concluded the letter by suggesting that colonists grow more hemp—a satirical punchline meaning he wanted more rope for hanging political dissidents.

But it wasn't just the elite talking about and growing hemp. In an era long before strong synthetic fibers, hemp was a valuable crop for anyone to cultivate. It wasn't unusual to find 12-foot-high hemp plants in the colonies. In 1774, county leaders in Virginia decreed that growing hemp should be encouraged and that to wear clothes made from American-grown hemp should be "considered as a Badge of Distinction and Respect, and true Patriotism."

Colonial governments accepted hemp as payment for taxes and paid subsidies to hemp farmers, in hopes of cutting reliance on foreign imports, especially from the world's leading hemp producer at the time, Russia. When the American Revolution began, the need became even more acute, as the colonists' naval operations relied on hemp-derived ropes and sails.

Throughout this period, hemp in the colonies also served

medicinal purposes. At the time, of course, no one had any understanding of the cannabinoids inside the hemp plant—namely CBD—but they did report positive effects. The most influential medical books in America, such as the 17th century *Anatomy of Melancholy* by Britain's Robert Burton, recommend hemp as a treatment for mental health issues. In the 18th century, *The New England Dispensatory* suggested hemp as a treatment for pain and inflammation, while *The Edinburgh New Dispensatory* recommended it as a cough remedy.

Although it was in the medical books and used as part of folk remedies, hemp wasn't especially popular for medical purposes in early America. That began to change in the 1830s, after an Irish physician working in India started experimenting with both marijuana and hemp as healing agents to treat muscle spasms, stomach cramps, and general pain. When word of William Brooke O'Shaughnessy's work spread, modern Western medicine began using cannabis more extensively, often in the form of tinctures taken by dropper. By 1890, a prominent British neurologist, Sir John Russell Reynolds, found hemp effective for tics, migraines, and asthma. The plant that had performed so well and for so long as an industrial staple seemed to have a bright future for widespread medicinal acceptance. Reynolds wrote in *The Lancet* that cannabis "when pure and administered carefully, is one of the most valuable medicines we possess."

Remember This: The hemp plant has long had important industrial uses, but it was also used for medicinal purposes in early America.

PROHIBITION

As the 20th century dawned, industrialization brought synthetic fibers that made hemp less necessary. New drugs, such as aspirin, emerged, and they had one major advantage. Treatment with cannabis, despite its effectiveness, always had brought the possibility of psychoactive effects, as hemp and marijuana were often intermingled, especially for medicinal purposes. Aspirin had no such issues—although other newly popular medications, including morphine and opium-derived drugs, certainly did. Nonetheless, cannabis's popularity began to fade.

66 My Take

I have been using a cream infused with CBD and vitamin E for my skin. I find it works about as well as my prednisone cream without requiring a prescription or having the possible side effect of thinning skin. —**Donna Harvey, RN, Key West, Florida**

99

Worried about the intoxicating effects of cannabis, and in the grips of a prohibitionist mind-set, state governments soon began criminalizing cannabis. While alcohol was made nationally illegal in 1920, Massachusetts passed a law restricting cannabis in 1911. Maine, Wyoming, and California followed with their own restrictions two years later and New York City soon after. Between 1915 and 1927, 10 states completely banned it. By 1937, all 48 states had passed laws to regulate and restrict cannabis to some degree.

During this period, Harry J. Anslinger, a virulent anti-cannabis crusader, became the first director of the Federal Bureau of Narcotics, an agency in the US Treasury Department established in response to the growing problems of opium and drug trafficking. Later generations would call this position "drug czar," and Anslinger boasted a longevity that any czar would envy. He served in his position from 1930 until 1962. Anslinger's anticannabis campaign succeeded in demonizing the plant, with no room for nuance to distinguish between marijuana and hemp strains. His contention was that cannabis causes madness and criminal behavior.

As many have noted, the policy may have been motivated by more than just an antipathy toward cannabis. The Mexican Revolution of 1910 had led to many Mexican refugees crossing the border into the United States. Some of the new arrivals brought with them a method of cannabis usage that had been relatively rare in the United States. They didn't bother with tinctures—they smoked it. Some members of the African-American community, engaged in their own migration northward, also had been smoking cannabis. Anslinger openly disdained Mexican-Americans and African-Americans. He began railing against the plant, using the Spanish nickname for cannabis—marihuana—which up until that time had been unknown in the United States. Anslinger used propaganda and the power of law to simultaneously vilify cannabis and minority populations that he detested.

In this environment, a church group financed a film aimed at parents to inform them of the purported dangers of their children smoking marijuana. The resulting 1936 movie—*Reefer*

Madness—featured crazed high school students overtaken by hallucinations and ultimately insanity as they engage in a variety of crimes. It was one of several anticannabis propaganda movies of the era.

By 1937, Congress had passed the "Marihuana Tax Act," which Anslinger had drafted. While the new law didn't technically criminalize marijuana or hemp on a federal level, it mandated that people who sell the flowers of the plant must register with the Internal Revenue Service, follow specific procedures, and pay a special tax. Just days after the law went into effect, Moses Baca, a 26-year-old from Mexico, was found with marijuana in a Denver rooming house and charged with not paying the marijuana tax. Baca was sentenced to 18 months at the federal penitentiary at Leavenworth and is often considered the first casualty of the US federal government's war on drugs. His dealer, a Colorado career criminal and former bootlegger named Samuel Caldwell, was also arrested in Denver and charged with selling marijuana. He was sentenced to four years at Leavenworth. At the sentencing, Judge John Foster Symes said, "I consider marijuana the worst of all narcotics, far worse than the use of morphine or cocaine. Under its influence, men become beasts. Marijuana destroys life itself. I have no sympathy with those who sell this weed." The process was complete. In just a few decades, cannabis had been transformed from a useful crop and beneficial remedy into a crime.

Thirty-three years later, President Richard Nixon made it official, signing the Comprehensive Drug Abuse Prevention and Control Act, which made cannabis fully illegal and classifying it as a Schedule 1 drug, a regulatory designation used for substances that have no medical value and high potential for abuse. Other Schedule 1 substances include heroin, LSD, and ecstasy. (Schedule 2 drugs, by contrast, are drugs that are considered to have at least some medical value. These include cocaine, methamphetamine, Ritalin, Adderall, and opioids such as oxycodone and Vicodin.)

Though a majority of states have legalized cannabis for at least medical purposes, on a federal level, it is still considered a Schedule 1 drug. One consequence: According to federal law, only one place in the United States—a University of Mississippi farm—can grow marijuana legally, and only for research purposes. Since potential researchers rely on federal grants and subsidies, this has had the effect of squelching almost all American research into cannabis for the past 50 years. The restriction affected marijuana and hemp equally—until December 2018 when the Farm Bill was signed into law. It wasn't until then that hemp finally broke free from its controversial sibling and was now fully legal under federal law.

> **Remember This:** For decades, hemp was effectively banned by the US federal government because of its association with marijuana, a designation that only ended in 2018.

BREAKTHROUGHS

In 1939, just two years after the federal government enacted the tax law that, in effect, criminalized cannabis, the US Treasury Department granted a prominent University of

Illinois chemist and researcher named Roger Adams a license to study the plant. (Anslinger was predictably opposed and spoke out against researching what he considered "the devil's lettuce.") But a year later, in 1940, Adams—a Harvard grad and descendant of President John Adams—first discovered cannabidiols in the cannabis plant. His contribution was significant—recognizing CBD and THC as unique chemical compounds and isolating them from the rest of the plant. But this was just a baby step. It wasn't clear to anyone, including Adams, which of the compounds produced the plant's various effects, from medicinal to psychoactive.

Researchers began testing these new discoveries. Some 1946 work by Walter S. Loewe found that THC caused a type of trance in mice and a "central exitant action" in rabbits, while CBD showed no observable effects on behavior. This was the first clue—mostly ignored at the time but obvious in retrospect—that THC had mood-altering psychoactive properties and CBD did not. But more than 15 years would pass before science understood the underlying chemical structures that would confirm it conclusively.

It was Israeli researcher Raphael Mechoulam, Ph.D., working in his lab at Hebrew University of Jerusalem, who searched the hardest. He knew scientists had earlier discovered and isolated the compounds that gave opium and the cocoa leaf their intoxicating properties. He wanted to do this for cannabis—to understand which parts caused which effects. Mechoulam succeeded, first describing the chemical structure of CBD in 1963 and THC in 1964. In the following years, he established the nonintoxicating, antioxidant nature of CBD and that it was

THC that produced the marijuana high. For these contributions, he is widely considered, in scientific circles, the father of modern cannabis.

After Mechoulam's breakthrough, cannabis research quickened (though not in the United States, where the full legal ban of all cannabis went into effect in 1970). By the mid 1970s, the first licensed cannabis tincture, most likely containing full-spectrum CBD, was released for medicinal purposes in the UK. In 1980, Mechoulam made another huge contribution, when he first studied the effect of CBD on epilepsy—early work that eventually led to the successful FDA-approved CBD drug, Epidiolex, which four decades later now provides incalculable relief to many epileptic patients.

It wasn't until the late 1980s that scientists began to identify and understand built-in CB-1 receptors in the brain and CB-2 receptors throughout the body, and how they interact with compounds from the cannabis plant. In 1990, molecular biologist Lisa Matsuda and her colleagues at the National Institute of Mental Health put the puzzle together, identifying the endocannabinoid system (ECS), a complex network that runs on the power of the body's naturally occurring internal cannabinoids but also responds to external cannabinoids (such as CBD and THC) from the cannabis plant. The ECS is responsible for keeping many key elements of the body in balance, including sleep, appetite, pain and stress tolerance, immunity, inflammation, and more. (For more on the ECS, see page 62.)

The folk remedy that had been used for centuries was now finally better understood. In a half century of fits and starts, scientists had discovered CBD and THC and figured out the basics of how they work inside the body. Experts were now able to clone the key receptors, allowing for more study and discoveries. In the history of science, this kind of watershed moment is usually followed by a flood of further research, each study building on the last until a sophisticated understanding emerges. With cannabis, however, this process was dramatically stunted by the unique legal constraints in the United States and elsewhere. Decades of potentially fruitful medicinal research was lost. For THC, in the United States, this federal prohibition persists. But for CBD, with enactment of the 2018 Farm Bill, which fully legalized the hemp strain of cannabis, the chains were finally unlocked, leaving many experts hoping that a golden age of new discoveries may be only beginning.

> **Remember This:** In the last 80 years, through a series of breakthroughs, science has slowly come to understand CBD and how it's matched remarkably well to the body's endocannabinoid system.

THE BOOM

Many people aren't waiting for new scientific discoveries. They're excited about CBD right now and are happy to be part of cannabidiol's emergence as a full-fledged phenomenon. Today, CBD has come out of the chemistry labs and into the mainstream, on a rocket. Because of its unique provenance—sibling to marijuana, banned by the government for so long, part of ancient healing remedies known by cultures around the world—CBD has a mystique that has helped fuel its rise.

And rise it has. Even just five years ago, the term CBD was more likely to refer to a town's central business district than a plant extract. In Peabody, Massachusetts, for decades CBD meant Christian Book Distributors, a large and successful local business serving bookstores everywhere. In 2019, after one too many callers asking what happened to their gummy bear order, the owners gave in, and changed the name of their family business to Christianbook.

Given the current hype and potential staying power of cannabidiol, it may have been a good move. Of the 2,616 respondents to the 2019 *Prevention* CBD survey, more than 95 percent said they were aware of CBD, with most of them saying they had heard about it from media coverage or friends, and others citing the now ubiquitous "CBD Sold Here" and other signs that have popped up nationwide almost overnight. Nearly three-quarters had either tried CBD or were interested in trying it, with pain, anxiety, inflammation, and insomnia as the leading reasons.

So far, cannabidiol enjoys a solid reputation. In a 2019 Harris Poll, among those familiar with CBD, 96 percent agreed that it should be available, with a large majority favoring no restrictions at all. More than three-quarters say it has at least some health benefits, with a third crediting CBD with "a lot of health benefits."

With its popularity growing so fast, it's hard to know exactly how many Americans are regularly using CBD, but it seems to be in the tens of millions. According to the 2019 Harris Poll and Cowen & Company market analysis, the number is 18 million, or 7 percent of all adults. Some estimates go even higher. The Harris Poll indicated that more than 45 million had at least tried CBD. According to 2019 *Consumer Reports* research, 26 percent of Americans had tried CBD in the previous two years—a number that translates to more than 65 million people.

In a mid-2019 Gallup poll, 14 percent of US adults said that they personally use CBD products, which represents more than 35 million adult Americans. By comparison, about 8 percent take fish oil, which has long been the most popular health supplement for its omega 3 fatty acids. Other natural supplements—such as melatonin, echinacea, garlic, and ginkgo biloba—are each used by about 1 percent of Americans or less. Just a couple of years after hitting the public consciousness, CBD already finds itself as the leading natural supplement. And its fans will tell you there's good reason. In the *Consumer Reports* research, about three-quarters of users said it helped ease symptoms and about half said it was extremely effective. In fact, 22 percent of users said that, for them, cannabidiol replaced a current medication, with more than a third saying that by using CBD they were able to give up taking an opioid, such as Percocet or oxycodone. (Also of note, about half gave up an over-the-counter medication, such as Advil or Tylenol.)

The ratio of CBD users is one in five among adults age 29 and younger, according to the Gallup poll. Geographically, CBD is most popular in the West, where 21 percent of respondents said they use CBD (compared to 11 percent in the East). As in the *Prevention, Consumer Reports*, and Harris surveys, the top reasons given are pain, anxiety, and insomnia.

According to business analysts, the number of users will only grow in the next several years. Cowen projects that the market will double multiple times in the next five years. In CBD circles this is considered a conservative estimate—as other firms have predicted even higher, faster growth.

The hype is real. And among the millions of CBD users out there, many celebrities have jumped on the trend, which, in turn, has only increased that hype. Beyond all the science and commerce fueling the CBD phenomenon, perhaps no day signified the boom of CBD more than April 27, 2019. On that afternoon, Kim Kardashian West, always in tune with the zeitgeist, rode the wave and increased the visibility for CBD by hosting what she called "my CBD baby shower." She offered her celebrity guests CBD vape pens and a chance to make their own CBD-infused bath oils and bath salts and shared images of the event with her nearly 150 million fans on Instagram. She had earlier told her followers, "Anyone that knows me knows that I am obsessed with CBD everything." In one post from the event, Kardashian says "Let's zen out for a Saturday. So everyone have a puff and put on some oil." She said she planned the CBD-themed celebration because she had been "freaking out so much" as an expectant mother with small children and wanted to relax. The story was picked up by media around the world, often with an explanatory accompanying story along the lines of "What Is CBD?"—an unlikely seminal moment in the popular rise of cannabidiol. (See page 108 for cautions about CBD and pregnancy.)

Among the famous, she's not alone. Whoopi Goldberg

believes in CBD enough to start her own CBD business, creating a menstrual cramps relief product (which also includes THC). Jennifer Aniston told *Us Weekly* "CBD helps with pain, stress, and anxiety. It has all the benefits of marijuana, without the high." Actress Olivia Wilde used CBD to help soothe her neck aches during a strenuous Broadway run. It was widely reported that Melissa McCarthy used CBD cream to prevent high-heel pain at an Academy Award ceremony—the same reason Mandy Moore used CBD at the Golden Globe awards. Morgan Freeman reportedly turned to cannabidiol (and THC) to relieve the ongoing pain stemming from a 2008 car accident. Martha Stewart advises Canopy Growth, a company that sells CBD for humans and pets. Michael J. Fox has advocated medical cannabis as a treatment for Parkinson's disease, and his foundation has lobbied for more funding for research into medical cannabis. Willie Nelson, never a stranger to cannabis, has introduced a line of CBD-infused coffee beans called Willie's Remedy.

In sports, like everywhere else, CBD and medical cannabis are gaining interest every day. Bubba Watson, one of the world's best professional golfers, is an outspoken fan and promoter of CBD, and at age 41, he has told reporters he thinks it could extend his career. NBA coach and former player Steve Kerr created some controversy when he mentioned in the media that he had used medical cannabis to help with chronic back pain. "I don't think it's a big deal," Kerr said in a press conference. "But I do find it ironic that if I said I used OxyContin for relief for my back pain, it would not have been a headline.

Having gone through a tough spell over the last year with my own recovery from back surgery, and a lot of pain, I had to do a lot of research. You get handed prescriptions for Vicodin, OxyContin, Percocet. . . . The stuff [opioids] is awful. The stuff is dangerous. The addiction possibility, what it can lead to, the long-term health risks . . ." While there are rules against cannabis use among NBA players, Kerr sees a change coming. "I think as the public gets more educated, and as people get more educated, there will ultimately be a policy that includes medicinal CBD, oils, whatever is best suited for pain."

Other sports are already moving in that direction. In late 2019, Major League Baseball removed CBD (and THC) from its banned list. USA Triathlon, that sport's national governing body, became the first organization of its type to sign a partnership agreement with a CBD company. Many elite triathletes had been afraid that using CBD for muscle pain might cause them to fail a drug test if the CBD product also included THC. USA Triathlon chose a Colorado company called Pure Spectrum because their CBD is backed by "strict third-party testing protocols to assure the products are pure."

In the celebrity medical field, CBD also has fans. Sanjay Gupta, M.D., who had previously been a skeptic of medical cannabis, helped legitimize cannabidiol with a landmark CNN 2013 special showing its potential for helping children with epilepsy—and the cruelty of a system that denied relief to suffering children due to outdated anticannabis laws. "I have sat in labs and personally analyzed the molecules in marijuana that have such potential but are also a source of intense controversy," he wrote in 2014, referring to CBD. "I have seen those molecules turned into medicine that has quelled epilepsy in a child and pain in a grown adult. I've seen it help a woman at the peak of her life to overcome the ravages of multiple sclerosis. I am more convinced than ever that it is irresponsible to not provide the best care we can, care that often may involve marijuana." Dr. Gupta received criticism from some, but his transformation was complete. "I am not backing down on medical marijuana," he said. "I'm doubling down."

> **Remember This:** In the last few years, CBD has become a phenomenon, embraced by celebrities and tens of millions of Americans.

LEGAL CONFUSION, THEN CLARITY

In the United States, the legal status of cannabis—both marijuana and its sister CBD—is an odd riddle. Currently, marijuana is illegal on a federal level, but legal in some states. Meanwhile, CBD is generally considered legal to possess and use on a federal level, but illegal in some states. For CBD fans, fortunately, that list of illegal states is tiny and likely getting smaller. Nebraska and South Dakota own the distinction as the last two states where CBD products are illegal (while in Idaho, regulations ban any CBD products that contain any THC, even if it's a trace amount under the federal limit of 0.3 percent). According to some expert predictions, those lagging legislatures are expected to eventually catch up with the rest of the country (Legal interpretations of CBD are still evolving. Check before buying.)

Since CBD is not approved as a food additive, some jurisdictions—including California, New York City, and Georgia—have banned it as an ingredient in foods, a position supported by the FDA. In fact, it's been reported that New York health inspectors have confiscated CBD-infused cookies.

On a federal level, since the signing of the Farm Bill in December 2018, it is legal to cultivate hemp (as long as it contains less than 0.3 percent THC). The law states that hemp-derived CBD specifically is no longer a controlled substance under the purview of the Drug Enforcement Administration (DEA). Hemp is now managed by the US Department of Agriculture (USDA) as a crop rather than by the Justice Department as an illegal substance.

66 My Take

For nearly eight years, I've suffered from chronic pain in various muscles. I've seen multiple specialists, but none have come up with any diagnosis nor any treatment beyond conventional general pain management. I was encouraged to try CBD. For a week before starting it, I decreased the other pain medications so as to give it a real test. I took a 20 milligrams capsule once per day for six days, and it had no effect at all. By that time the pain was so bad that I gave up on CBD and went back to the other medications. **—Nina G., Old Saybrook, Connecticut** 99

But for months after passage of the Farm Bill, confusion reigned, with states failing to clarify their cannabis laws. After some prominent cases, state laws changed to allow virtually all CBD products to be legal. In a 2019 police raid in the Dallas suburb of Duncanville, Texas, police broke down the door of a tobacco shop, seizing CBD products, including bath balms and lollipops. After the media got involved, charges were not pursued. Soon after, a new Texas law made CBD legal as long as it contains less than 0.3 percent THC.

Meanwhile, in Florida, at a checkpoint for Disney World, Hester Jordan Burkhalter, a great-grandmother who said she had been planning her Disney visit for two years, was arrested when a county deputy found CBD oil in her purse. According to media reports, Burkhalter was using the CBD for arthritis on the advice of her doctor. "I have really bad arthritis in my legs, in my arms, and in my shoulder," she said. "I use (CBD) for the pain because it helps." She was even carrying a note from her physician, but at a time of cannabis confusion in the legal system, it didn't matter. Burkhalter was shocked at her arrest. "I've never had one speeding ticket in my life," she said. The authorities stood firm, releasing a statement that said, "This was a lawful arrest, as possession of CBD oil is currently a felony under Florida State Statute and deputies are responsible for enforcing Florida law and Orange County ordinances." Weeks later, Florida clarified the law, making CBD legal as long as its THC level is kept under 0.3 percent. Charges were dropped.

Remember This: After years of bans and confusion, CBD is legal in almost every state. The US federal government legalized hemp in 2018, which makes CBD legal on a federal level.

HOW IT WORKS

WHERE CBD COMES FROM, HOW IT AFFECTS OUR BODIES, PLUS COMMON MISCONCEPTIONS AND THE TRUTHS YOU SHOULD KNOW.

What cannabidiol is and how it works in the body is a complex topic that science is just starting to understand. Even experts who've devoted their lives to the study of the subject have trouble fully explaining the processes and mechanisms at work and why CBD has the effect that it does.

Fortunately, this is not a textbook and there will be no exam. On these pages, don't expect dizzying descriptions of complex physiological responses and theories that require a medical degree to decipher. Instead, this book takes a different tack. First, it's helpful to understand the basic science of CBD so you can feel informed. This knowledge may help guide you if you decide to delve deeper into the world of cannabidiol. Or it just may make you sound smart the next time you're talking to friends, family, or colleagues and the subject of CBD arises, as it often does these days. One common thread of such conversations: misconceptions about cannabidiol. To help you see through the fog and enhance your understanding of this much-discussed plant extract, this chapter is devoted to five things you should know about CBD, plus three common CBD myths.

Later, Chapter 4 provides practical advice to help you understand how CBD works with various conditions. Chapter 5 is a useful guide to various product types of CBD, with the best wisdom for being a smart consumer.

66 My Take

I have a patch of psoriasis on my head that appeared a couple of years ago. I was really distressed with it so my daughter drove me an hour from my home to a health food store that sells CBD cream. It cost over $45 for a 2 ounce jar. In addition to cannabidiol, ingredients include: "coconut oil, water, beeswax, and essential oils of juniper berry lavender, rosemary, blue tansy, and hellichysm." This jar says it contains 200 milligrams of cannabidiol (CBD). The short story is that is does nothing for my skin condition. A little vaseline does just as much. I have put it on other skin problems on my face, and it is just another oil. This product is an expensive ripoff!

—**Jane VomSteeg, Diamond Springs, California**

99

5 THINGS YOU SHOULD KNOW ABOUT CBD

At this early stage of its development, how CBD interacts with the body and its effects are not fully known. Too many questions remain unanswered—to be decided through years of future lab study and clinical observation. Still, there are plenty of important things to understand—about the cannabis plant, how CBD works in your body, where it comes from, and what comes along with it.

THE PLANT

Cannabidiol is extracted from the cannabis plant—formally known as *Cannabis sativa* L—which has various strains. As described in Chapter 1, the longtime star of the cannabis family is called marijuana, known for its psychoactive effects brought on by the compound THC, which is found in the plant's flowers. It is widely grown in greenhouses and other controlled environments to maximize its yield of potent flower.

Its sibling strain, called hemp, or industrial hemp, is much more workmanlike, known for its commercial uses. Its seeds and stalks have long been used in many products. The Dutch painter and printmaker Rembrandt sketched his drawings on paper made from hemp, and European shipbuilders centuries ago used it to make sails. It's a tall, sturdy plant that is grown like other agricultural crops in an open field. It can do well in a variety of regions. China produces more hemp than any other country.

In good conditions, a hemp plant can grow to a foot high in just three or four weeks. At full maturation, it can be 15 feet or taller. Contrary to a common misconception, hemp is not the male version of the female marijuana plant. For both marijuana and hemp, it is the female plant that is cultivated and harvested, ideally before it is fertilized by the male pollen. As the hemp flower (or bud) reaches full bloom, it secretes certain cannabinoids and resin to attract the pollen from the male plants and produce seeds. This secretion is where CBD comes from.

Another misconception is that CBD is the medicinal part of the cannabis plant, while THC is the recreational part. It doesn't work that way. Both THC and CBD, which are found in various strains of the cannabis plant, have medicinal qualities. They can work well together, but also apart. Both compounds are found in marijuana, while hemp features little or no THC. Today, to be legally considered hemp, a plant must contain less than 0.3 percent of THC, which is about 30 times less than even a weak marijuana plant. Almost all marijuana plants have CBD but no legal hemp plants have more than a tiny trace amount of THC.

THE ENDOCANNABINOID SYSTEM

In the 1990s, scientists—led by Lisa Matsuda, Ph.D., at the National Institute of Mental Health—were trying to figure out why marijuana gets people high. As part of their research, they discovered the endocannabinoid system (ECS), an internal network that had never been understood before. Its job inside the body of all animals is to use neurotransmitters to maintain a stable internal environment for health, mood, temperature, pain modulation, and more.

This system has receptors within the cells of the intestines, liver, pancreas, reproductive organs, and bones, as well as the brain and central nervous system. (The ones located in the brain and central nervous system are called CB1 receptors. The ones in the organs and elsewhere in the body are CB2 receptors.) Every day, enzymes within the human body create billions of beneficial natural chemicals that bind to these receptors, which helps keep the body well regulated and on an even keel. That's the main purpose of the ECS—to keep your body in a stable state of homeostasis. But while the enzymes produce these chemicals all day long, scientists believe they also reappear to destroy those same chemicals, creating the need for more. There is no storage—the body is constantly using and destroying these natural chemicals. It's a never-ending cycle.

This discovery was amazing enough. But what really astounded the scientists was figuring out how substances in the cannabis plant could play a positive role with these receptors—in the brain and body. As described in Chapters 1 and 2, within cannabis are compounds known as cannabinoids that, according to the scientists, mimic or improve the performance of these internal chemicals in a remarkable way and play a key role to boost this cellular system. These cannabinoids, including CBD, had been discovered decades earlier but were not fully understood. Without them, the body is forever depleting and restoring those beneficial enzymes that keep the system stable. But scientists began to understand that by consuming CBD, the system may be disrupted, stopping the depletion and allowing the benefits to linger.

The naming of the endocannabinoid system underscored the connection between plant and animal. Scientists named the newly discovered system after the cannabinoids that they had earlier found in cannabis. For the new system, they added a prefix, "endo," that means "internal". The beneficial chemicals that bind naturally to those receptors around the body were dubbed endocannabinoids, while the ones that come from plants, such as CBD, received the prefix, "phyto" meaning "relating to plants" and became phytocannabinoids.

The effect of this signaling system on the body and brain is wide and deep. "The ECS helps us to eat, sleep, relax, forget what we don't need to remember, and protect our body from harm," says Jahan Marcu, Ph.D., of the International Research Center on Cannabis and Mental Health in New York City. It's a natural mechanism that helps the body deal with stresses, including extreme exercise. "We always thought the 'runner's high' was due to the release of dopamine and endorphins," says Joseph Maroon, M.D., clinical professor and vice chairman of neurosurgery at the University of Pittsburgh Medical Center. "But now we know the euphoria is also from an endocannabinoid called anandamide."

While that's an example of an internally produced endocannabinoid, the most famous of the plant-based phytocannabinoids is THC, which causes the psycoactive effects of marijuana by binding with those CB1 receptors in the brain, where there are more CB1 receptors than even opioid receptors.

CBD doesn't bind to the receptors themselves. Rather, it improves their performance, probably by allowing the body's natural production of key enzymes to keep going without their otherwise inevitable self-destruction. This positive effect occurs in CB1 receptors in the brain as well as in the CB2 receptors throughout the body, which is one reason so many people are excited by the potential of CBD. Unlike THC, which primarily affects the brain, CBD promises a body and brain benefit. While science has yet to figure out all the details, it is known that the ECS affects almost every physiological process, including sleep, hunger, mood, pain, inflammation, the nervous system, and memory. For this reason, the hope is that the phytocannabinoid CBD can bring relief for many conditions, though much human study is still needed to prove the case.

HOW CBD IS MADE

Yes, the CBD found in products comes from the hemp plant, but how? It begins with the growing and harvesting of hemp plants that have been cultivated to contain a high amount of CBD and almost no THC. The amount of cannabinoid in various hemp varieties can vary widely, but CBD growers use the type of hemp that produces the most CBD. Since hemp is a field crop, generally planted in high numbers, the plants are usually harvested using a combine harvester—a huge piece of machinery well known on farms for simultaneously reaping, threshing, and winnowing crops. Once harvested, the extraction process begins, with the aim to separate and collect the essential oils and compounds from the flower of the hemp plant. It can be done with a variety of extraction solvents; the cleanest involves a nontoxic fluid form of carbon dioxide that is used extensively by the food industry. The FDA gives the process GRAS categorization, meaning "generally regarded as safe."

The solvent is forced through the plant, pulling out the CBD, essential oils, lipids, and other compounds. At this point, the solvent and any other undesirable elements are removed by filtration, leaving an oil that is naturally high in CBD. (For more about the extraction process and how it impacts CBD products, see page 137.) To further purify it, the product is heated—a process known as *decarboxylation*—which transforms the cannabinoids into a form that's ready to interact with the body's cannabinoid receptors. The oil can then be used in a wide variety of products.

The most popular type of products are tinctures. In the 2019 *Prevention* survey of CBD users, 57 percent said they used them. A tincture is a tiny, concentrated drop of CBD oil that goes under the tongue, where mucous membranes quickly absorb it, bypassing the digestive system and liver to reach the bloodstream fast. The CBD is whisked to the carotid artery and directly to the brain's endocannabinoid receptors. The elapsed time between taking the drop and feeling any effects can be as little as 15 minutes or less, depending on the dose.

Tinctures are the most common way to take CBD, but not the only way. In the 2019 *Prevention* survey, 35 percent of CBD users said they applied topical lotions, balms, or patches, and 21 percent had ingested their CBD through chewable gummy candies. For 19 percent of users, vaping oil was their delivery method, while 13 percent took capsules. (For a helpful, detailed guide to each of these product types, see Chapter 5.)

ALL ABOUT TERPENES

Spend enough time poking into the world of CBD and soon you'll come across a word that you may not have encountered before: terpenes. Unless your interest runs heavily to botany, you may not know that these natural compounds found in the essential oil of plants may play an important role within the cannabis plant and ultimately, if you ingest CBD, within your body. As with all parts of the endocannabinoid system, much still needs to be learned about the effects of terpenes, especially when combined with phtyocannabinoids such as CBD. But for consumers of CBD, terpenes are an important element to understand.

Science knows there are many types of terpenes, found in herbs, fruits, and other plants. In cannabis they ooze from the sticky resin glands, the same glands that produce CBD, THC, and other cannabinoids. Among their duties: to provide plants with their aroma and flavor. When you smell a fragrant pine tree, you're smelling terpenes. Marijuana plants are steeped with many terpenes and have the fragrance to prove it. Hemp, which is generally considered nonaromatic with little flavor, has fewer terpenes, but many believe it's still enough to have an effect in the body.

One major example is myrcene, which is the most common terpene in cannabis. In some cases, more than half of the terpenes within a hemp plant may be myrcene. It's also found in lemon-grass, which has long been used in folk remedies, as well as in hops (giving beer its distinct aromas). In marijuana plants, the myrcene level plays a role in whether the plant is considered "indica" (producing a more relaxing high) or "sativa" (producing a more uplifting high). Plants with more myrcene terpenes tend to be classified as the relaxing indica strain, and studies with rodents have shown that myrcene does produce a sedating effect. This leads some experts to speculate that when CBD users report calming and sleep-inducing benefits, myrcene from within the hemp plant may be contributing to that effect. But the study of CBD is new enough that many of these questions are still unanswered. Is it the cannabidiol itself that calms you? Or is it the myrcene within the plant? Or is it a mix of the two, and if so, what's the perfect combination? Science still isn't sure.

And with dozens of terpenes to study, the possibilities are vast. For instance, another cannabis terpene, linalool (which is found in lavender, too), is also purported to produce relaxing effects. And then there's caryophyllene, which is found in black pepper and many herbs and spices, as well as in cannabis. Caryophyllene is a unique terpene in that it's the only one that has the ability to act like a cannabinoid, binding to the CB2 receptors in the body's organs, where, some believe, it may work through the endocannabinoid system to provide anti-inflammatory benefits. Again, no one knows for sure how all these ingredients work together, which is one reason most CBD users hedge their bets and buy "broad-spectrum" CBD that comes combined with terpenes, too.

THE ENTOURAGE EFFECT

In some products CBD is presented in its most independent form, known as "CBD isolate." In these cases, everything else the hemp plant offers is stripped away. A CBD isolate means there's 0 percent of THC and no other cannabinoids. Isolate often comes as a powder to be used for homemade CBD products and also can be found in oils, edibles, capsules, and other products.

But while solo CBD may sound ideal, many people believe there's a better way. They put forth the theory that CBD is more effective when it arrives in your body accompanied by terpenes and other natural parts of its native plant. After all, they reason, CBD is just one of many active compounds and beneficial ingredients in cannabis. And while hemp doesn't have all the compounds found in other strains (most notably, it does not produce THC), it still has more than 100 cannabinoids and other ingredients, including helpful fatty acids, vitamins, proteins, and terpenes.

These proponents also believe that when interacting together in a synergistic way, CBD and other components of cannabis produce a stronger effect than any of the single ingredients could on their own. In other words, one plus one equals three. They call this "the entourage effect." When shopping for CBD, you will often see the phrase "full spectrum," "whole spectrum," or "broad spectrum." These marketing terms mean the product is promising that the CBD won't come solo but rather will ride with its whole helpful crew. (The difference between the terms? Full- or whole-spectrum products usually feature everything from the hemp plant, including trace amounts of THC, while broad-spectrum products have undergone an extra step to ensure that all THC is removed. For more details, see page 141.)

Most researchers consider the entourage theory plausible, but as with all things CBD, they want to see more research before getting fully on board. For some, the idea of the entourage effect only muddies the waters of their exploration—it's harder to study the effectiveness of CBD if its true power only comes when combined with hundreds of other ingredients. Some, however, give some credence to the general concept. They point to medical marijuana as an example of the ultimate entourage effect. When pure synthetic THC first became available in the 1980s, some thought it might provide the same medicinal effects as the full cannabis flower. But patients reported more relief from full-flower, whole-spectrum products. It became clear to many that dozens of the other cannabinoids and ingredients in cannabis—including CBD—were working in conjunction with the THC to produce medicinal results.

In fact, some experts believe—putting aside legalities and psychoactive effects—that CBD seems most effective when it's teamed with a full range of terpenes and cannabinoids, including a hefty dose of THC. After all, they say, marijuana (including THC, CBD, and many other cannabinoids and terpenes) has been used as a healing substance for centuries by various cultures. Today, new strains of medical marijuana are being bred and marketed with even more CBD in the mix. (While marijuana strains traditionally might be, say, 18 percent THC and less than 1 percent CBD, new medicinal products are now popular in dispensaries at all kinds of THC:CBD ratios, including 1:1.) And fans are reporting relief for pain, anxiety, and sleeplessness from such products.

For people who hold a state-sanctioned medical marijuana card or live in a state where marijuana is fully legal, these kinds of products may be an option. However, they come with complications, most notably psychoactive effects and the certainty that you won't pass a drug test. With broad-spectrum CBD, which includes many of the potentially beneficial side ingredients but no THC, there are none of those complications.

While it's accepted that CBD plays a role in medical marijuana, the question is, how effective is CBD when the THC isn't there? Does cannabidiol keep its medicinal profile when it's on its own or teamed with only the nonpsychoactive elements of its native plant?

Early testing has shown that full-spectrum CBD seems to have a more sustained effect than isolates and may provide a wider medicinal potential within the body. But for experts, more research is warranted to understand how these different ingredients work together and which combinations are best for various conditions and effects. In the meantime, since other parts of the hemp plant are safe and considered generally beneficial, the consensus for those interested in CBD is that it's a good idea to shop for broad-spectrum products.

> **Remember This:** CBD is a natural, plant-based compound and when bought in broad-spectrum form, comes with a variety of other beneficial ingredients.

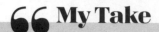 **My Take**

I sought out CBD oil for the fatigue, body pain, sleep deprivation, and anxiety I was experiencing living with stage IV metastatic breast cancer. My hope was to receive relief from the side effects I was experiencing from my meds and the disease. I heard CBD could help with my pain, and I bought some from a local store, but did not receive the results I was looking for.

I later found a producer that manufactured their own products from organic Wisconsin hemp. I decided to purchase from this manufacturer after getting a full understanding of how they process the CBD oil through their unique extraction methods, allowing them to get the greatest benefit from the hemp. I started using the new product and felt the effects of it almost immediately!

I've continued using the CBD oil and it allows me to enjoy a good quality of life while living with a terminal illness, which is priceless! I have no derogatory interactions with my meds. I am pain free. I have achieved a level of calmness and I sleep well. I've also used CBD body balm and lotion to eliminate any areas of inflammation when it appears. I have experienced a better quality of life since I've incorporated CBD oil into my daily wellness program. I encourage anyone seeking the benefits of CBD oil into their wellness program to research what is available before running to their local market and buying any CBD oil off the shelf.

—Linda Lambrecht, Mosinee, Wisconsin

THREE CBD MYTHS

With the outlaw history of cannabis (detailed in Chapter 2) and the scientific mysteries of cannabinoids, it's easy to see why CBD is subject to misunderstandings and misconceptions. Add in a zealous CBD industry making all kinds of promises and critics spreading ill-informed objections, and it's easy for wrong-headed notions to take root. Here, we take a look at three stubborn ones and clear the air.

MYTH I: TAKING CBD COULD GET ME IN TROUBLE.

Some people worry that CBD might cause them to fail a drug test. The truth is, drug tests only measure one cannabinoid from the cannabis plant—the psychoactive compound THC. (To be precise, tests look for a compound created by the body when it metabolizes THC.) One thing drug tests don't measure is the amount of CBD in your system. By definition, the THC level in cannabidiol is less than one third of 1 percent—just a trace at most, which is much less than could ever cause a failed drug test.

It's kind of like drinking a nonalcoholic beer, which often contains less than one half of 1 percent of alcohol by volume, while a regular beer might contain 4 to 6 percent. Yes, there may be tiny amounts of alcohol in the nonalcoholic product, but not nearly enough to cause inebriation or a failed sobriety test, unless someone drinks dozens of bottles in the same sitting. Similarly, marijuana is often 15 percent THC or more, which means it may contain more than 50 times the amount of THC than what is the top limit for CBD products. It's likely you would need to ingest thousands or tens of thousands of milligrams of CBD to fail a drug test—much more than almost anyone would ever use at one time.

But remember, there is no FDA control over the ingredients in a CBD product. As discussed on page 37, studies have repeatedly shown that the bottle sometimes contains surprises. In most cases, the discrepancies revealed in those studies involved mislabeling the amount of CBD in the product (sometimes it was more than what was on the label; sometimes less.) But in some cases, a full-spectrum CBD product contained a little too much of the spectrum—including levels of THC that are above the magic 0.3 percent cutoff. In an often-quoted study published in *JAMA*, researchers bought CBD online and found that 18 of the 84 samples tested contained detectable levels of THC, at levels as high as 6.43 mg/ml (still less than what a typical marijuana user would likely consume, but far more than what CBD products are supposed to have.)

This can cause problems, especially for CBD users who face drug tests as part of their employment. In 2019, a Phoenix woman named Tammy Allen, who had been taking CBD that she bought online to help with her seizures and migraines, told ABC News, "I tested positive for THC, and I ended up being put on administrative leave." Eventually, Allen said she lost her job due to the violation. She was told that after the test, her employers believed she had recently smoked marijuana. While many share the fear of the same fate, among the millions currently using CBD, such cases are relatively rare.

In addition to some incidence of mislabeled products, there's also potential variability in how THC is measured. First, the 0.3 percent is based on the dry weight of the cannabis plant, not the finished CBD product. Plus, each state has its own way of figuring this number. (Some collect the top 6 inches of the plant, others collect more or less.) And there's no uniformity on testing for THC in finished products. This raises the possibility of THC unexpectedly appearing where it shouldn't be. But experts suggest the chances are low.

Confusion about CBD can also cause problems for travelers. In May 2019, Lena Bartula, a 71-year-old grandmother, was arrested at Dallas/Fort Worth International Airport when CBD oil was found in her travel bag after she arrived from Mexico. Bartula, who said she relied on the CBD for the aches and pains of aging, was handcuffed and jailed for two nights on felony drug charges. The charges were eventually dropped, and Texas law was later clarified to allow CBD. If there had been more than traces of THC in her oil, however, the outcome may have been much worse. Meanwhile, the Transportation Security Administration (TSA) changed its policies in 2019 to allow passengers to travel with CBD products. But if the CBD somehow contains more than the critical 0.3 percent THC, such legal protections disappear—which means, it pays to know what's in your bottle.

To improve your odds, experts suggest buying from reputable companies, the kind whose websites post the product's "certificate of analysis" (showing the exact purported amounts of CBD and THC, as well as how it was tested.) Some users who are especially concerned about drug testing only buy CBD isolate. This is cannabidiol in its purest form, which makes contamination by THC extremely unlikely (For more on this, see page 142.) For other helpful tips for buying CBD safely, see Chapter 5.

MYTH 2: TAKING CBD IS RISKY.

Some people wonder if cannabidiol is safe for long-term use. Others question whether it will affect their mind and get them high or worry that it's addictive. Since CBD is newly popular, some fear unforeseen drug interactions or side effects.

The reality is that even experts who don't advocate cannabidiol generally consider it remarkably safe. At common doses it is considered nontoxic, although the FDA says there is limited data so there could be risk. That said, with only trace amounts of THC, it doesn't cause a psychoactive high. And no one has died from overdosing on any cannabis product.

But fears remain. A 2019 Harris Poll found that a third of Americans are concerned about how CBD interacts with prescription drugs. While many users haven't reported any serious problems with CBD drug interactions, there are some important cautions to note. The National Library of Medicine recommends not taking it with the seizure medication clobazam (Onfi and Sympazan) since CBD may slow the liver's work to break down the drug, which could change the effect of the drug or cause side effects. With another seizure medication, valproic acid (Depakene), CBD is not recommended because it could cause liver injury.

For some sedatives, it's a good idea to check with your doctor to ensure that CBD's interaction with the drug doesn't cause too much sleepiness. In fact, some experts recommend checking with your doctor before starting CBD if you're using any drug that is broken down and changed by the liver, which includes more than half of the pharmaceuticals on the market, everything from ibuprofen to Prevacid to Paxil to Xanax. Taking CBD with these drugs may change the effects and side effects of the medication. More studies are needed to fully understand these interactions.

There are many health experts who believe cannabidiol is completely safe, no matter what the dose. Even an incredibly huge dose such as 5,000 milligrams a day will not damage vital organs, says Jahan Marcu, a pharmacological expert. Overall, the World Health Organization has stated, "there is no evidence of public health related problems associated with the use of pure CBD."

At the same time, experts are looking closely at the plant extract's effect on the liver, especially at extremely high doses. A study by the University of Arkansas found that after ingesting high doses of CBD, mice experienced liver damage and in some cases died as a result in just a few days. In fact, as part of the clinical trials for the CBD epilepsy drug Epidiolex, researchers discovered liver toxicity in some patients, with 5 to 20 percent experiencing some kind of liver issue. "The FDA identified certain safety risks, including the potential for liver injury," the agency concluded. It's important to note that Epidiolex treatments contain a megadose of CBD that's much higher than what's typically used by other CBD users. While the National Institutes of Health (NIH) notes that such liver injury is rare, more study is currently underway, and doctors do monitor liver enzymes when using Epidiolex to treat children.

NIH researcher and endocannabinoid expert Pal Pacher, M.D., Ph.D., is leery of much of the positive hype around CBD, but liver damage is one thing he doesn't worry much about. He says many common over-the-counter medications have the same risk, and for CBD, the only amounts that have caused any problems are so big that for the average user, they would be what he calls "nonsense doses."

In the Harris Poll, 38 percent of Americans said they were concerned that CBD might have unknown side effects. As with any plant extract, CBD affects each body differently. Some people feel nothing at all—no side effects, no positive benefits. In those cases, proponents often suggest experimenting with higher doses. If that doesn't work, the most painful side effect may be financial more than physical. At as much as $60 or more for a 500 milligram tincture bottle, CBD isn't cheap.

Other people experience a variety of effects, including, in some cases, unwanted symptoms. According to the NIH, side effects can include dry mouth, low blood pressure, lightheadedness, and drowsiness. (In cases where CBD is being taken to help with insomnia, that sleepiness, of course, switches from side effect to desired effect.) Others have experienced headaches, irritability, diarrhea, nausea, decreased appetite, red eyes, hunger, rashes, or in a positive twist, euphoria. Since CBD is unregulated, some of these reported effects may have come from other substances incorrectly marked CBD. In any case, according to a 2018 study published in *Cannabis and Cannabinoid Research*, one in three CBD users had experienced an unexpected effect. "I'm reasonably certain new kinds of side effects will emerge," says J. Michael Bostwick, M.D., a psychiatrist at the Mayo Clinic. To date, however, most of cannabidiol's unexpected effects have been minor and relatively rare.

One effect no one should worry about, according to experts, is addiction. "In humans, CBD exhibits no effects indicative of any abuse or dependence potential," says the World Health Organization. This is often seen as one of CBD's potential strengths. Unlike opioids and other pharmaceuticals, which often bring the high risk of potentially disastrous addiction, experts say CBD may provide relief without that danger.

The biggest risk of CBD may be taking it instead of a medication that you need. "Misleading and false claims associated with CBD products may lead consumers to put off getting important medical care, such as proper diagnosis, treatment, and supportive care," the FDA has warned. The agency has cited CBD companies for claiming that it can treat serious diseases such as cancer, Alzheimer's disease, and diabetes. Such claims are not backed by verifiable evidence.

MYTH 3: CBD IS A WONDER DRUG.

By standard pharmaceutical definitions, cannabidiol is not even a drug at all. It's a plant extract—a naturally occurring compound. For many people, this is a major part of the appeal. CBD's fast rise in popularity has brought hope and excitement that there's now a natural, nonaddictive solution for a wide variety of issues, with no serious side effects—what some might call a wonder drug. For others, this all seems a bit too good to be true. They are skeptical about the lack of indisputable human research and dubious of the hype.

Such skeptics point to the beauty industry, which, based largely on the anti-inflammatory promise of CBD, now markets cannabidiol as if it is some kind of miracle elixir. CBD has become a featured ingredient in moisturizers, shampoos, conditioners, mascaras, soaps, antiwrinkle serums, antiacne formulas, muscle rubs, sleeping masks, face lotions, body creams, and more.

The fiercest CBD advocates believe there's almost nothing cannabidiol can't help. There are even products that feature CBD in tampons—to help treat menstrual cramps. Online it's easy to find CBD touted as a treatment for brain cancer, lung cancer, breast cancer, leukemia, heart disease, Crohn's disease, Alzheimer's, autism, ALS, neuropathic pain, obesity, obsessive compulsive disorder, schizophrenia, and much more. For much of the serious medical community, these claims are problematic.

"I don't have a problem until it is hurting someone," says Dr. Pacher, NIH investigator and past president of the International Cannabinoid Research Society, a medical organization of professionals devoted to the study of medicinal cannabis. "People can take CBD and I don't care. They may spend lots of money for it, but it won't induce harm. But there are so many unsupported claims. For example, there is zero human evidence that it is working to treat cancer patients. But I worry about desperate people giving up chemotherapy thinking that CBD could help them. I have a problem with that, because many of these people may die and their best chance right now, chemotherapy, will be lost because of false hope."

Dr. Pacher compares the CBD boom to the hype around resveratrol and red wine two decades ago. This compound found in grapes was first isolated in 1939 (almost the exact same time that the compound cannabidiol was first discovered in the cannabis plant). Sixty years later, it gained enormous popularity, spurred by some intriguing research suggesting that perhaps the compound could reduce inflammation, help fight cancer, and improve longevity. The ingredient was heavily marketed and pharmaceutical companies poured money into research. Resveratrol appeared in more than 20,000 research papers in the past 20 years and was studied in more than 130 clinical trials. But it was found to be poorly absorbed when taken and never gained acceptance in the medical community. The product is still available as a niche supplement, and some advocates still believe in its power. The hype, however, is over.

"There were lots of benefits attributed to red wine," Dr. Pacher says. "Resveratrol was seen as the key ingredient in red wine, much like CBD is seen as the key medicinal ingredient in medical marijuana. But for resveratrol, that was speculation. And with CBD, it's not so simple, either. We know that cannabis has medicinal effects, but there's no proof that CBD is the medicinal part. There are terpenes and other minor cannabinoids, plus THC. At the time, you could buy resveratrol everywhere and people were taking it for everything. It was overhyped. It was the new magic bullet to prevent aging. And ultimately, in my view, it was a deception."

Complicating the issue today, according to Dr. Pacher, are unscrupulous CBD companies who are trying to profit on the boom, with some having little knowledge of their own products. "There is lots of money involved. Billions of dollars. And some of these companies, they make claims, but they have no idea," says Dr. Pacher, who has coauthored more than 300 peer-reviewed publications and has been a part of the NIH since 2003. "It's kind of the wild, wild West."

In the normal life cycle of a new medication, research and development is followed by clinical trials, a patent, government approvals, and finally marketing to the public. But because CBD is a natural part of a plant that anyone can access, cannabidiol itself cannot be patented. What is proprietary for a company are the delivery vehicles (oils, creams, and more) and the sourcing and extraction of their cannabis. This is one of the things that has made CBD a grassroots sensation. To many, it is the underdog health product that comes from nature, not from a lab. While many advocates love this about CBD, it does allow irresponsible companies into the industry, which means consumers need to be especially vigilant about product quality. Even within the best companies, results can be difficult to predict and standardization is hard to achieve since the main ingredient is a plant compound rather than a man-made formula.

Further research will ultimately define the scope of cannabidiol's full benefits. A common expectation among experts is that it will be useful for some issues and some people, but not a panacea by any means. Whether it's a wonder drug depends on your perspective. For the epilepsy sufferers and their families who have gone from hundreds of seizures a day to zero, CBD feels like a miracle. For an anxiety, insomnia, or pain sufferer who finds that CBD works well enough that they can stop using opioids or other heavy medication, CBD may seem like a natural wonder. For someone expecting that it will solve all their health problems instantly, that's unlikely.

"CBD is not a scam," Yasmin Hurd, director of the Addiction Institute of Mount Sinai Hospital, told the *New York Times,* after leading a study of 42 recovering heroin addicts and finding that CBD reduced cravings and anxiety. "It has potential medicinal value, but when we're putting it into mascara and putting it into tampons, for God's sake, to me, that's a scam."

> **Remember This:** Lots of people love the effect they receive from CBD, but it's unlikely to provide a magic bullet for most serious conditions. It's also unlikely to cause you to fail a drug test, get addicted, or endure any significant side effects.

GOOD FOR WHAT AILS YOU?

WHAT SCIENCE AND EXPERIENCED USERS SAY ABOUT THE EFFECTS OF CBD ON SPECIFIC CONDITIONS.

--- **IN THIS CHAPTER** ---

Fair Warning
Conditions and Care
CBD and Pets

Trained healers and ordinary people have been using the cannabis plant as a treatment for a wide range of purposes for thousands for years. It was listed as an anesthetic in a Chinese book of medicinal plants that has survived since the year 100. In ancient India, cannabis preparations were prescribed for insomnia, headaches, and pain. In the 19th century, cannabis was an ingredient in popular patent medicines sold in the United States and Europe as remedies for headaches, stomach cramps, muscle pain, and other common ailments.

Meanwhile, scientists in recent years have documented the effectiveness of many medicinal plants long used as folk remedies. Published studies have shown, for instance, that ginger relieves nausea and indigestion and white willow bark has been proven to be an effective analgesic. The 80-plus years of prohibition in the United States on growing and processing cannabis prevented or strictly limited research into its potential use as a treatment for any condition. Studies, however, continued in other countries, some with lab animals as subjects, some with humans. Now new research reports about the effects of CBD for specific conditions are being published by researchers in the United States and around the world.

In this chapter, you'll find out about studies that give credence to the experiences CBD users are reporting and get insights into how the cannabinoid may be affecting their bodies and symptoms. Before looking at what the research says, though, it's important to remember a few critical facts.

FAIR WARNING

In 2017, the National Academy of Sciences (NAS) published "The Health Effects of Cannabis and Cannabinoids: The Current State of Evidence and Recommendations," a wide-ranging review of the research to that point. It made four conclusive statements.

For adults with chemotherapy-induced nausea and vomiting, oral cannabinoids are effective anti-emetics [substances that control nausea].

In adults with chronic pain, patients who were treated with cannabis or cannabinoids are more likely to experience a clinically significant reduction in pain symptoms.

In adults with multiple sclerosis (MS)-related spasticity, short-term use of oral cannabinoids improves patient-reported spasticity symptoms.

For these conditions the effects of cannabinoids are modest; for all other conditions evaluated there is inadequate information to assess their effects.

The findings of the NAS carry a lot of weight in the scientific community, but it is the FDA's responsibility to regulate the marketplace for health and wellness products in the United States. As of 2020, the FDA has approved only one CBD formula for treatment of only one condition. Epidiolex, a CBD-based oral solution, may be prescribed for the treatment of seizures associated with two rare and severe forms of epilepsy, Lennox-Gastaut syndrome and Dravet syndrome, in patients two years of age and older. (It is the first drug of any kind approved by the FDA for the treatment of patients with Dravet syndrome.)

In a 2019 public statement, the FDA set parameters around the sale of CBD products, declaring it illegal to market CBD by adding it to a food or labeling it as a dietary supplement. And CBD products may not be labeled or marketed as a cure for any specific health problems. You should be wary of any product that does make such a claim.

While the FDA is protecting American consumers, the World Health Organization (WHO) studied the risks of CBD use and announced its results in a 2018 report: "CBD exhibits no effects indicative of any abuse or dependence potential ... there is no evidence of public health related problems associated with the use of pure CBD." For those reasons, the WHO Expert Committee on Drug Dependence recommended that CBD not be classified internationally as a controlled substance. In other words, the organization stated that CBD should not be treated as a medication with a high potential for abuse.

The conclusions from the WHO report are widely accepted even by experts who are skeptical about CBD: It is not likely to be abused and it's generally safe for anyone to use. Researchers and CBD users have observed few side effects, which include drowsiness, dry mouth, and diarrhea for some people taking it orally. Still, there are a few cautions to consider before trying it. Most important, CBD may hamper the effectiveness of some prescription drugs—in particular, it appears to interfere with certain medicines that act as anticoagulants or anticonvulsants used to treat seizures. Further, CBD is processed through the liver, so people with liver problems should be especially careful about using it. Regardless of your condition, you should discuss using CBD with your health-care providers before trying it.

Among the most pressing issues for researchers is determining the right dosages for particular people and problems. Right now, most CBD users are relying on the trial and adjustment approach to finding the appropriate dose for themselves. Bryan Doner, D.O., chief medical officer of Compassionate Certification Centers, a medical cannabis health-care provider in Pittsburgh, Pennsylvania, proposes a simple dosage formula as a starting point for any of his patients: 0.5 milligrams of CBD for every kilogram (2.2 pounds) of body weight for oral doses. (For a 150-pound person, that works out to about 35 milligrams.) He recommends dividing the daily total amount into two separate doses—morning and evening. Dr. Doner advises starting with lower doses of inhaled CBD. Topical treatments may need higher concentrations of CBD to be effective.

Age, condition, and experience with cannabis use can all have an effect on how CBD impacts you. That's why Dr. Doner advocates for the "low and slow" approach. What this means is that patients should always start off with a lower dose and then slowly increase in increments of 5 milligrams. He has observed that underdosing is a common problem for people new to CBD. "Patients tell us they don't feel any effects," he says, "so we tell them to gradually increase the dose until they do feel it."

CONDITIONS AND CARE

In this section, you'll find references to laboratory and clinical studies that showed CBD treatment provided benefits to a specific (often small) group of test subjects suffering from defined symptoms. Please bear in mind that none of the research conclusively establishes that CBD is an effective treatment for any condition (other than for seizures caused by two kinds of epilepsy) nor is there any reliable determination about how or how much CBD to take to treat any problem. There are no prescriptions here. The science simply doesn't support those kinds of recommendations. Instead, this chapter can be used as a helpful guide to CBD's potential for a wide range of conditions, featuring the most compelling research and possible CBD treatment options.

"Prior to going to the store to purchase any CBD-containing product, consumers should consider researching CBD and cross-referencing their findings with whatever disease or ailment they are concerned with," Richard Carmona, M.D., former surgeon general of the United States, told *US News and World Report*. To help you get started, we quote a lot of research reports from peer-reviewed medical journals in this section so you can see what the scientists are saying about their results. (See the list of studies in the Resources section on page 168.)

ADD/ADHD

Attention deficit disorder (ADD) and attention deficit hyperactivity disorder (ADHD) refer to a range of symptoms that include difficulty with concentration, impulsive behavior, and constant fidgeting. It primarily affects children, though 3 percent of adults deal with the symptoms on a daily basis. Many sufferers and the caregivers of children with these challenges are using CBD to help calm minds and relieve anxiety.

Research says: A group of 30 adults with ADHD were given either Sativex, a pharmaceutical oral spray that includes THC as well as CBD, or a placebo, in a study published in the *Journal of the European College of Neuropsychopharmacology*. The results were inconclusive, but the researchers did observe "a nominally significant improvement in hyperactivity/impulsivity and a cognitive measure of inhibition, and a trend towards improvement for inattention." That may offer promise to the many people using or considering CBD to help manage the symptoms of ADHD, but more and larger studies are needed to determine if there are meaningful benefits.

CBD's potential: Among people with ADD/ADHD, cannabidiol was reported to be most helpful "with staying on task, minimizing distractibility, and mitigating agitation or irritability," according to a 2019 survey by Project CBD, a nonprofit promoting research into the medical uses of CBD. The cannabinoid "appears less effective at minimizing the tendency to lose things and procrastinate (common to ADD/ADHD) and sometimes made those symptoms worse."

CBD treatment options: Those seeking all-day symptom management go for oral doses of capsules, tablets, or chewables because the CBD is released gradually. For immediate relief from acute episodes, you can choose more rapidly absorbed tinctures or oral sprays.

Caution: Do not give CBD in any format to children living with ADD or ADHD before consulting their health-care providers. CBD may interfere with the effects of other medications or aggravate specific symptoms.

Related conditions: Oppositional defiant disorder, conduct disorder, learning disorders, anxiety, depression

ADDICTION

CBD alone won't break the grip of cravings for opioids, alcohol, and nicotine, but it is being used to help ease the symptoms of withdrawal for many who are trying to quit their addictions. Early studies indicate it might help reduce relapses among serious drug abusers and aid tobacco users who are trying to decrease their consumption.

Research says: It took just a single 800 milligram dose of CBD to reduce the craving for heroin among addicts participating in a study published in *Neurotherapeutics*. The effects were prolonged, "lasting two or more weeks after administration," the researchers state. "The ability of CBD to inhibit relapse behavior was still apparent weeks after the last exposure, suggesting that CBD could impact the course of heroin dependence even following a potential lapse condition after a period of abstinence."

Researchers in the UK studied the effects of CBD on 24 cigarette smokers. The participants were given "CBD inhalers" to use whenever they felt an urge for a cigarette. "The main finding of this study was a dramatic reduction in the number of cigarettes smoked across a 7-day period in the individuals using the CBD inhaler, compared to no reduction in the placebo group," the scientists reported.

CBD's potential: Pain, anxiety, and insomnia are common causes of substance abuse and they are symptoms that CBD is often used to treat. The cannabinoid also helps control nausea, which tends to accompany withdrawal from opioids.

CBD treatment options: Tinctures, oral sprays, and vaporizing may provide a fast-acting response to the discomforts that incite cravings. Oral doses via capsules and tablets twice or three times daily maintain steady levels of CBD in the body, which are believed to be helpful for controlling pain and anxiety.

Related conditions: Abuse of alcohol, tobacco, or narcotics; anxiety; depression

ANXIETY

About 40 million adults in the United States age 18 and older (about 19 percent of the population) live with anxiety and related disorders, making it the most common mental health problem, according to the National Institute of Mental Health. Veterans and others who have endured traumatic events are especially vulnerable to debilitating anxiety. Anxiety disorders are characterized by excessive nervousness, fear, apprehension, and worry that is out of proportion to the actual danger. Physical symptoms include nervousness, tension, panic, increased heart rate, sweating, fatigue, and trouble concentrating. Easing these types of symptoms is one of the main reasons for trying CBD.

Research says: When patients with generalized social anxiety disorder were given an oral dose of 400 milligrams of CBD, they reported "significantly decreased anxiety" versus a group of control subjects, according to a study published in the *Journal of Psychopharmacology.* The researchers conducting the study also used neuroimaging to measure blood flow in different parts of the subjects' brains. The results suggest that "CBD reduces anxiety and that this is related to its effects on activity in limbic and paralimbic brain areas."

Another group of scientists surveyed all of the available research on CBD and PTSD and shared their findings in the journal *Frontiers in Neuroscience.* They conclude that "Human and animal studies suggest that CBD may offer therapeutic benefits for disorders related to inappropriate responses to traumatic memories. The effects of CBD on the different stages of aversive memory processing make this compound a candidate pharmacological adjunct to psychological therapies for PTSD."

CBD's potential: The brain areas responsible for managing heart rate, blood pressure, and other responses to stress have a high concentration of cannabinoid receptors. By activating those receptors, CBD is believed to trigger the release of hormones and enzymes that soothe stress reactions.

CBD treatment options: People who experience periodic panic attacks and other acute symptoms of anxiety often rely on the fast absorption and action that results from inhaling vaporized CBD oil. For those trying to maintain a healthy balance all day long, taking capsules or other slow-release oral products two or three times a day may provide more consistent, longer-lasting effects.

Related conditions: Panic disorder, post-traumatic stress disorder, social anxiety disorder (social phobia), obsessive-compulsive disorder

ARTHRITIS

The daily pain of stiff, swollen joints hampers the regular activities of about one in five people. Older people are especially prone to osteoarthritis, the result of deteriorating cartilage that begins in middle age. Rheumatoid arthritis is an autoimmune disorder that causes painful swelling in the joints. It affects children as well as adults. CBD's reputation as an anti-inflammatory treatment has made it popular for both short-term and long-term relief among arthritis sufferers.

Research says: "Transdermal administration of CBD has long-lasting therapeutic effects without psychoactive side effects," say researchers who studied lab animals with the symptoms of arthritis in a report in the *European Journal of Pain*. "Thus, use of topical CBD has potential as effective treatment of arthritic symptomatology."

CBD's potential: Cytokines are proteins that are secreted by immune system cells. They trigger the responses to injury or illness that cause inflammation. Endocannabinoids disable the cytokines when their work is done, preventing the persistent inflammation that causes joint pain.

CBD treatment options: CBD balm or lotion applied directly onto swollen joints are designed to bring quick relief directly to the pain spot. Twice daily oral doses of CBD fortify the whole body to protect it against autoimmune reactions.

Related conditions: Rheumatism, psoriatic arthritis, osteo-arthritis, autoimmune disorders

AUTOIMMUNE DISORDERS

This term covers a wide range of conditions that are linked because they cause the immune system to attack healthy tissue. Rheumatoid arthritis, lupus, inflammatory bowel disease, multiple sclerosis, and psoriasis are among the most common. People with these chronic problems are trying CBD to relieve the pain, swelling, and rashes that come with these conditions.

Research says: "Cannabidiol reduces spasticity, pain, inflammation, fatigue, and depression in people with multiple sclerosis," state researchers in a report in *Frontiers in Neurology*.

The scientists also observed reduced use of opiates and other pain relievers among MS sufferers who took CBD.

CBD's potential: The common factor among these disorders is chronic, unwarranted inflammation, which is regulated by the endocannabinoid system. CBD is also believed to slow down T-cell production and suppresses immune system memory, which could decrease the likelihood of future autoimmune attacks.

CBD treatment options: Proponents believe oral doses two or three times daily would have the best chance of keeping the immune system supplied with cannabinoids to control symptoms. Topical creams and balms applied to the surface of skin may help soothe rashes and other kinds of outbreaks.

Related conditions: Crohn's disease, inflammatory bowel disease, lupus, multiple sclerosis, psoriasis, psoriatic arthritis, rheumatoid arthritis, and many others

CHRONIC PAIN

Serious injuries, surgery, disease, and muscular and nervous system ailments can cause pain that is persistent and long-lasting. Opioid drugs are commonly prescribed for people suffering from daily pain, but those medications come with unwelcome side effects, and they can be addicting. CBD has become an appealing alternative for those seeking relief.

Research says: Results of a study of CBD's effects on rats and inflammation was published in the journal *Pain*. "Acute, transient joint inflammation was reduced by local CBD treatment," the scientists reported. "Prophylactic administration of

CBD prevented the development of [induced] joint pain at later time points." While this study of laboratory animals can be encouraging to people seeking relief from chronic pain, research with humans is needed to determine if CBD reduces and prevents inflammation in people.

CBD's potential: TRPV, the technical abbreviation for transient receptor potential cation channel subfamily V, is a key link in the nervous system's communication chain that brings pain sensations to the brain. CBD binds to TRPV1, which suggests it can influence pain perception.

CBD treatment options: CBD users are treating "hot spots" of pain with topical applications of CBD balm or lotion to get quick, direct relief to those places. Oral doses, in many cases two or three times a day, are the typical choice for relief from aches throughout the body.

Related conditions: Post-injury or surgical pain, cancer, neuropathy

DIABETES

The two types of diabetes have similar symptoms, but somewhat different causes. Type 1 is an autoimmune disorder caused by the destruction of insulin-generating beta cells in the pancreas. It prevents the body from safely managing blood sugar levels. People with Type 2 diabetes are also unable to produce sufficient insulin as needed because of factors such as diet, obesity, and activity level. The symptoms of both types include fatigue, blurred vision, slow healing cuts and bruises, chronic thirst, and tingling, pain, or numbness in the hands and feet. Almost

10 percent of people in the United States have one of the two types of diabetes. It is a complex, life-threatening condition and needs to be treated under the care of a doctor. Type 1 can't be avoided by taking CBD or any lifestyle change. Researchers are, however, exploring whether CBD can help control the causes and alleviate the symptoms of Type 2.

Research says: Treatments tested on laboratory animals such as mice and rats always need further evaluation in humans, but the results of a study of obese mice treated with CBD, published in the medical journal *Autoimmunity*, were intriguing. Only 30 percent of obese mice given CBD developed diabetes versus 86 percent of a control group, report researchers. "Our results indicate that CBD can inhibit and delay destructive insulitis," the scientists state. In another small study, 62 human subjects with non-insulin-treated Type 2 diabetes were given CBD, another treatment, or a placebo. The researchers report in the journal *Diabetes Care* that "compared with baseline (but not placebo)," CBD decreased resistin and increased glucose-dependent insulinotropic peptide, two hormones that play a critical role in our body's insulin management.

CBD's potential: Much more evidence than these two very limited studies have produced will be needed before it's clear whether CBD has any benefits for people with Type 2 diabetes.

CBD treatment options: Diabetes is a complex, life-threatening condition that should be treated under the care of a physician. Consult your doctor before trying CBD in any form..

Related conditions: Metabolic syndrome, neuropathy, retinopathy

EATING DISORDERS

The causes of anorexia, bulimia, and binge eating are complex so it is unlikely that CBD alone would cure them. However, researchers are beginning to investigate if it can help manage its symptoms, which include anxiety, stress, and, for some patients, a disruption of normal appetite.

Research says: In 2018, the Center for Medicinal Cannabis Research (CMCR) at the University of California (UC) San Diego School of Medicine announced plans to study CBD as a treatment for anxiety associated with anorexia nervosa in adult patients. "Anorexia nervosa is difficult to treat and, in some cases, may be a fatal condition," said Emily Gray, M.D., clinical assistant professor of psychiatry, in a press release from the university. "There is preliminary research that suggests cannabinoids may be beneficial in treating this and other eating disorders. The administration of CBD is of interest because of the possibility that this drug might reduce anxiety and perhaps normalize reward and motivation."

CBD's potential: The use of CBD to control anxiety and its related symptoms is the primary reason why researchers believe it may be beneficial for people with eating disorders. The endocannabinoid system also manages two hormones, ghrelin and leptin, which play a central role in controlling appetite and feeling satisfied when eating. This might make CBD useful for people who are trying to gain control of excessive eating.

CBD treatment options: Oral spray, tincture, or vapor are rapidly absorbed so they may offer quick help in high-stress situations. Capsules, tablets, or other ingestible products have longer-lasting effects but are better not taken on an empty stomach.

Related conditions: Anorexia, bulimia, binge-eating disorders

FIBROMYALGIA

The causes and mechanisms of fibromyalgia are not fully understood, but the symptoms are. They include chronic joint pain, headaches, anxiety, and trouble sleeping—the problems for which CBD is a popular treatment.

Research says: The studies of cannabis treatments for fibromyalgia patients specifically have so far included both THC and CBD, not CBD alone. Still, the results are encouraging. "We observe significant improvement of symptoms of [fibromyalgia] in patients using cannabis," report researchers at the Human Pharmacology and Neurosciences Unit, Institut de Recerca Hospital del Mar in Barcelona, Spain. "The present results seem to indicate a possible role of cannabinoids on the treatment of [fibromyalgia], although it should be confirmed in further clinical trials."

CBD's potential: CBD seems to reduce brain inflammation, which is linked to the pain and brain fog that afflict fibromyalgia patients. The endocannabinoid system also manages the body's response to stress, which often triggers outbreaks of fibromyalgia symptoms.

CBD treatment options: Edibles or other forms of oral doses gradually release CBD to the whole body. Topical applications such as creams and balms are formulated to treat pain in specific spots. For an all-over topical treatment, the CBD in bath bombs is absorbed through the skin while you soak in soothing warm water.

Related conditions: Autoimmune disorders, chronic fatigue syndrome, hyperthyroid syndrome, migraine headaches

INSOMNIA

Common problems such as pain and anxiety can disrupt healthy sleeping patterns for many people, but daily stress, hormonal changes, irregular work schedules, and lots of other causes can keep us up at night, too. CBD has become a welcome alternative to prescription and over-the-counter sleeping pills. CBD users report that it works quickly to get them back to sleep and it doesn't leave them feeling groggy the next day. In a national survey by *Consumer Reports*, about 10 percent of Americans who reported trying CBD said they used it to help them sleep, and a majority of those people said it worked.

Research says: "Cannabinoids could improve sleep quality, decrease sleep disturbances, and decrease sleep onset latency," conclude the authors of a review of published studies of CBD and sleep in the journal *Experimental and Clinical Psychopharmacology*. One of the studies found that subjects with insomnia taking 160 milligrams of CBD before bed slept longer and more deeply than those who had taken a placebo. (The study also found that lower doses of 40 milligrams and 80 milligrams of CBD were not effective.)

CBD's potential: Cannabinoid receptors in the brain are thought to be directly connected to the mechanisms managing the body's sleep/wake cycle.

CBD treatment options: Users who suffer from chronic

insomnia often take oral doses of CBD before bedtime. Those who have trouble going back to sleep find relief from rapidly absorbed vaporized CBD oil or sublingual drops.

Caution: In at least one study subjects reported that sleeplessness improved in the first month of taking CBD daily, but the benefits faded during the following months. This suggests CBD's ability to improve sleep may diminish the longer you use it. Other studies have not shown the same drop-off in effects.

Related conditions: Restless legs syndrome

MENOPAUSE

During the transition to and experience of menopause, women typically live with symptoms that include sleep disruption, pain and inflammation, anxiety, and hot flashes. Menopausal women are turning CBD to help moderate these daily discomforts.

Research says: No published studies have assessed the impact of CBD on menopause specifically, but "many of my patients report that it helps with sleeping and anxiety," says Lauren Streicher, M.D., clinical professor of obstetrics and gynecology at the Northwestern University Medicine Center for Menopause. "I've also seen some evidence CBD may influence bone metabolism, but at this time it is not a treatment for osteopenia or osteoporosis.

"There is currently no scientific data that CBD makes any difference with hot flashes beyond a short-term placebo effect," Dr. Streicher adds.

CBD's potential: The endocannabinoid system is involved

in regulating hormone activity as well as body temperature, so some experts theorize that it could relieve symptoms caused by rapid changes in hormone levels. Serotonin, a hormone that manages mood and can ward off depression, is also linked to the endocannabinoid system.

CBD treatment options: Sublingual strips and tinctures dissolve quickly through the membranes in the mouth and release CBD into the system, which may help bring fast relief when the discomforts are acute. Be aware, Dr. Streicher emphasizes, that the metabolism of menopausal women is altered and they may experience a "delay in the onset of action. I recommend that menopausal women who are trying CBD stick to low to moderate doses."

Related conditions: Perimenopause

MENSTRUAL CYCLES

For so many women, their monthly periods and the days leading up to them bring a variety of discomforts, including painful cramping, bloating, sleep disruptions, and anxiety. CBD has become a popular treatment for women seeking a natural remedy for these symptoms and many are reporting that "CBD appears to be highly effective in addressing mood and pain issues associated with female hormonal cycles," according to a 2019 study by the nonprofit Project CBD.

Research says: "There are many anecdotal reports that CBD helps with the symptoms that come with periods or premenstrual syndrome, but we don't have any conclusive evidence in the scientific literature," says Dr. Streicher, the professor of obstetrics and gynecology and also a member of the Prevention Medical Advisory Board.

CBD's potential: "I tell my patients that they can try CBD if they wish and it might be helpful," Dr. Streicher says, "though it is possible that many of the women who are touting it may be experiencing a placebo effect."

CBD treatment options: Topical preparations, such as balms and lotions, applied directly to pain spots may help relieve inflammation and the discomforts it causes.

Related conditions: Premenstrual syndrome

NAUSEA AND APPETITE

One of the first medical applications of cannabinoids was to help restore the appetites of cancer patients undergoing chemotherapy. That led to the development of synthetic THC medications, such as Marinol. More recently, people experiencing chronic nausea or loss of appetite have been turning to CBD for the same purposes. (Pregnant women should see page 108 before considering using CBD for any symptom.)

Research says: "CBD effectively prevented conditioned retching," report researchers in the *British Journal of Pharmacology (BJP)*. "Preclinical research indicates that cannabinoids, including CBD, may be effective clinically for treating both nausea and vomiting produced by chemotherapy or other therapeutic treatments."

CBD's potential: "The blockade of one subtype of receptor, the 5-HT3 receptor, could suppress the acute emetic response (retching and vomiting)," according to the same article in the *BJP*.

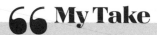 **My Take**

CBD treatment options: Sublingual drops or inhaled vaporized CBD oil are absorbed quickly, so they may be able to bring fast relief to acute nausea without causing further digestive distress.

Related conditions: Cancer treatments, motion sickness, and chronic nausea

OSTEOPOROSIS

Approximately 30 percent of postmenopausal women in the United States experience gradual decline in the density and strength of their bones, the condition known as osteoporosis. It leads to an increased risk of bone fractures, as well as back pain and imbalanced posture. We found no research so far on

CBD as a treatment for it, but scientists have linked the endocannabinoid system to skeletal development and maintenance.

Research says: "Our recent studies in mice and humans suggest an important role for the endocannabinoid system in the regulation of skeletal remodeling and the consequent implications on bone mass and biomechanical function," says a report in the *British Journal of Pharmacology*. They note that CB2 cannabinoid receptors are present in bone cells and that malfunctioning of a key gene involved in production of those receptors appears in analyses of people suffering from osteoporosis. (Read about the different types of receptors and their functions on page 63.)

CBD's potential: Osteoblasts and osteoclasts are two unique types of cells that play a primary role in building and maintaining our bones. Scientists have observed that these cells produce key endocannabinoids (anandamide and 2-arachidonoylglycerol) and the CB2 cannabinoid receptors they attach to. Research indicates that the activation of these CB2 receptors slows bone loss and encourages new bone formation. CBD's link to the CB2 receptors might make it useful in protecting against osteoporosis.

CBD treatment options: Swallowing a CBD capsule or tablet each day provides a constant supply of the cannabinoid for the body to use as needed.

Related conditions: Autoimmune disorders, including type 1 diabetes, rheumatoid arthritis, lupus, and hyperthyroidism, all increase the risk of osteoporosis.

PARKINSON'S DISEASE

A progressive nervous system disorder, Parkinson's disease affects movement, leading to tremors, rigid muscles, difficulty with walking normally, limited facial expressions, and trouble speaking and writing. Chronic pain, anxiety, trouble sleeping, and hallucinations or delusions are common symptoms as the disease advances. Researchers and caregivers are trying CBD to help alleviate some of these difficult-to-treat symptoms.

Research says: Hallucinations and delusions were reduced in Parkinson's patients who do not suffer from dementia after taking CBD capsules for a week, according to a study published in the *Journal of Psychopharmacology*. Another group of researchers, who reported their findings in the *Journal of Clinical Pharmacy and Therapeutics*, documented improvement in sleep quality, including fewer nightmares, among a small group of Parkinson's patients after taking a single dose of CBD.

CBD's potential: CBD acts as an antioxidant that scientists theorize provides protection against the rapid deterioration of neurons, which is a contributing factor to Parkinson's disease. The cannabinoid is also a popular treatment for anxiety and pain, two of the disease's most persistent symptoms.

CBD treatment options: Edibles, such as gummy bears or chocolate bars, are an appealing way to get Parkinson's patients to take daily doses of CBD.

Related conditions: Supranuclear palsy, multiple system atrophy, Lewy body disease, anxiety, sleep troubles

PREGNANCY

The discomforts of pregnancy and postpartum recovery often include pain and inflammation, nausea, trouble sleeping, and anxiety, the symptoms commonly treated with CBD. When seeking relief from these everyday problems, many women believe that a natural, plant-based remedy like CBD is safer for them and their baby than over-the-counter medicines.

Research says: "We definitively know that cannabinoids cross the placenta and are found in breast milk. And there have been credible published reports in the medical literature of problems with fetal growth and development related to the use of cannabis," says Dr, Streicher. Dr. Streicher, as well as the American College of Obstetrics and Gynecology, stress that pregnant women and those who are breast-feeding should not use CBD under any circumstances.

CBD's potential: Pregnancy is not the time to use CBD.

SEIZURES

As we explained earlier in this chapter, the FDA has approved a CBD-based drug for treatment of people with either of two rare and severe forms of epilepsy, Lennox-Gastaut syndrome (LGS) and Dravet syndrome. LGS is usually diagnosed in children ages 2 to 8 years old, and Dravet syndrome typically begins in the first 18 months of life. The medications that are typically prescribed to control seizures in people with other forms of epilepsy have not been effective for these patients.

Research says: Several research teams at different locations participated in clinical trials of CBD as a treatment for children with Dravet syndrome and LGS. These double-blind, placebo-controlled trials (the highest standard for medical research into treatments) were the first such studies of CBD in the United States. For the patients in the study suffering from Dravet syndrome, seizures were reduced by 39 percent in children treated with CBD versus a reduction of only 16 percent in the placebo group. "That's a modest difference, but statistically significant," says Elaine C. Wirrell, M.D., a consultant in pediatric neurology at the Mayo Clinic in Rochester, Minnesota, one of the institutions that participated in the study.

"The results of these studies demonstrate that, at a dosage of 20 [milligrams per kilogram of body weight per day], CBD added on to pre-existing [antiepileptic drug] treatment is superior to placebo in reducing the frequency of convulsive seizures in patients with Dravet syndrome, and the frequency of drop seizures in patients with Lennox-Gastaut syndrome. In the latter patients, a dosage of 10 milligrams/kilogram/day treatment was also superior to placebo," according to a report in the *Journal of Epilepsy Research*.

Bear in mind that these two specific types of epilepsy affect a small portion of the estimated 4 percent of people who suffer from epilepsy. CBD also helped control seizures among people with the more common forms of epilepsy in a small study published in the US-based journal *Pediatric Neurology*.

Seizures are a common symptom of epilepsy, but about one in every hundred people will have seizures in their lifetimes that are unrelated to the condition. The symptoms can include temporary confusion, a staring spell, uncontrolled jerking of arms and legs, loss of consciousness, and sudden rapid eye movement.

CBD's potential: Seizures appear to be related to inflammation in the brain, which may be reduced by CBD. The endocannabinoid system also triggers the receptors for GABA (gamma-aminobutyric acid), a neurotransmitter that calms excited neurons, particularly those related to motor control. Researchers can't say definitively how Epidiolex works, but it appears to use different pathways in the nervous system than other epilepsy drugs. One theory is that CBD regulates the amount of calcium inside of nerve cells. Too much calcium causes them to fire electric pulses too fast, leading to an overload in the brain. CBD may help maintain a healthy balance of calcium in nerve cells.

CBD treatment options: The prescription for the approved drug, Epidiolex, has substantially more CBD than the standard dosage recommendation we shared earlier in this chapter. It calls for 2.5 milligrams for every kilogram of body weight (or about 180 milligrams for a 160-pound person) each day for one week, increasing to 5 milligrams per kilogram for maintenance. Oil or tincture are the most frequently cited forms for using CBD to control seizures in the online discussion group hosted by the Epilepsy Foundation (epilepsy.com). For both prescriptions and self-treatment, the doses are typically spread out over two or three times of the day.

Caution: In the studies that led to FDA approval of Epidiolex, the subjects took CBD in conjunction with other seizure control medications. Talk to your physician about your antiseizure medications before trying CBD.

Related conditions: Epilepsy, sleep apnea and narcolepsy (another sleep related condition), Tourette's syndrome, and migraines are other conditions that may cause occasional seizures.

SKIN DISORDERS

Skin that is chronically itchy, dry, flaky, crusty, blistering, oozing, or reddened can be a source of both physical and emotional discomfort for people of all ages. These conditions can also lead to open sores and persistent infections. There are many causes of these conditions, from allergic reactions to autoimmune disorders. Patients report that CBD is proving helpful for relief from both the underlying causes and the visible symptoms.

Research says: Test subjects were provided with CBD-enriched ointment and instructed to apply it to lesioned skin areas twice daily, according to a report in *Journal of the American Academy of Dermatology*. The treated areas showed significant improvement based on skin evaluations by the researchers, and the subjects reported an 86 percent improvement in itching.

CBD's potential: Mast cells are immune cells that release histamine when activated, which leads to intense itching and inflammation. The endocannabinoid system directs the activation of mast cells.

CBD treatment options: Topical applications of CBD balms or creams are used to treat the outbreaks on the skin's surface. Daily doses of capsules or tablets may work to prevent the inflammation and release of histamines that trigger appearance of the symptoms.

Related conditions: Acne, eczema, inflammatory skin disease, pruritis

WOMEN'S SEXUAL HEALTH

Women of all ages and various medical conditions experience vaginal dryness, pain during sex, and orgasmic dysfunction. CBD oil applied topically acts as a "vasodilator," meaning it expands blood vessels and increases blood flow. That has encouraged women to try it as a treatment for these discomforts.

Research says: No high-quality research has demonstrated that CBD improves sexual response in women, but Dr. Streicher, author of the bestselling book *Sex Rx*, has suggested topical CBD treatments to her patients to increase vaginal lubrication and orgasmic function. "I tell my patients, especially diabetics who have small vessel disease and clitoral neuropathy to try it," she says.

CBD's potential: "Clitoral neurons and vaginal lubrication depend on capillary action, so CBD's function as a vasodilator may improve blood flow and sensation to their genitals," Dr. Streicher says.

CBD treatment options: Topical treatments, such as lotions or lubricants infused with CBD, are the most effective way to increase blood flow in the areas where it can help relieve discomfort and increase sensation.

> **Remember This:** Before you take CBD for any condition, consult with your physician about its benefits and risks for you.

CBD AND PETS

Dogs and cats are like four-legged family members, so their well-being tends to get as much attention as that of the rest of the household. And pets suffer from many of the same hard-to-treat health problems that humans do, including chronic pain, anxiety, seizures, and trouble sleeping. What's more, dogs and cats have an endocannabinoid system, just as we do. That's encouraged pet owners to try treating their animals with CBD, and many report that it has helped in a variety of ways.

Be aware that California is the only state so far to permit veterinarians to discuss the therapeutic use of cannabis-derived supplements for animals, though bills are pending in other states. But pet owners around the country are asking about it, according to a 2019 poll by the Veterinary Information Network (an online community for professionals). Nearly 30 percent (of the more than 2,000 vets who participated in the poll) reported that they are questioned about CBD for animals at least once a week by pet owners. Fifty-six percent of the vets acknowledge that they have had clinical experience with CBD products for dogs. And a solid majority believe it is beneficial: Fifty-six percent indicated that CBD products were somewhat helpful for chronic pain in their patients and 66 percent said they found CBD somewhat helpful for anxiety in pets. Most reassuring, 80 percent of the vets reported no side effects in pets except for mild sedation.

RESEARCH SAYS

Research into treating pets with CBD is just beginning—there's even less known about its effects on these animals than there is on people—so nearly all of the information about it is anecdotal. However, two ongoing (and as yet unpublished studies) do offer some support for giving pets CBD.

Dogs suffering from epilepsy received doses of CBD oil in a trial by Stephanie McGrath, D.V.M., a neurologist and assistant professor at Colorado State University's College of Veterinary Medicine and Biomedical Sciences. She reported that the canines had an 89 percent reduction in the frequency of seizures. "Overall, what we found seems very promising," Dr. McGrath said.

Dogs experiencing pain from osteoarthritis were given CBD as part of a study at the Cornell University College of Veterinary Medicine. The researchers noted that 80 percent of those taking CBD showed "significant improvement in pain levels and quality of life without discernible side effects."

CONDITIONS AND USES

Pain: Aging and injuries can leave pets with chronic discomfort, limited mobility, and reduced activity. Pet owners who have treated pets in pain are saying they are seeing the animals perk up and regain their energy and vitality. That's far from conclusive evidence, but it's interesting to note because dogs obviously aren't subject to the placebo effect (although their owners are). In a way, this observed improvement may be quite telling about what CBD can really do because the patient isn't aware of the treatment.

Anxiety: Whether because of unfamiliar situations, fireworks and other loud noises, traveling, visiting the vet, predisposition, and other reasons, both dogs and cats can experience intense stress and persistent anxiety. Many pet owners are reporting that CBD calms anxious animals. Horses are also prone to anxiety, so their owners are trying CBD for those symptoms and saying that it's soothing even for large animals.

Seizures: Epilepsy afflicts dogs and cats with symptoms similar to those that humans endure, including seizures. Animals may also be struck with seizures for other reasons, such as low blood sugar or brain and nervous system disorders. The research at Colorado State University and the experience of pet owners offers hope that CBD can help to reduce the frequency of the seizures.

Appetite: The National Institutes of Health has acknowledged that cannabinoids act as an antiemetic, helping to ease symptoms of nausea or vomiting, for people. When medications, illness, motion sickness, or other conditions cause pets to vomit repeatedly or to lose their appetite, pet owners are trying CBD to help.

SAFE TREATMENT

Just as with people, determining safe, effective CBD dosage levels for pets is a challenge. A good starting point is 0.5 milligrams of oral CBD for every kilogram (2.2 pounds) of the animal's body weight, says Angie Krause, D.V.M., who has a veterinary practice in Boulder, Colorado. (For a 20-pound dog, that works out to about 4.5 milligrams per dose.) Dr. Krause suggests trying small amounts first to gauge pets' reaction before giving them full-size, regular doses. Breaking up the total dosage into two separate servings—morning and evening—is also recommended.

You'll find CBD in all kinds of products for pets such as crunchy or chewy treats infused with CBD, flavored drops, pet-grade peanut butter, and coconut oil infused with CBD. You can also go with a basic CBD tincture, which you can squirt right onto your pet's tongue or onto a favorite food. "You can buy dog treats containing CBD, but the best form to administer is an oil or tincture," according to Jerry Klein, DVM, chief veterinary officer of the American Kennel Club. "This way, you can adjust your dog's dose drop by drop."

CBD oil drops squirted under an animal's tongue will be absorbed fastest. Of course, that's not always possible with pets. So, adding the drops to treats or regular meals works, too, but the CBD is absorbed more slowly and its effects are more gradual since it goes through the digestive system. Though there is no published research on topical CBD treatments for pets, you can find CBD balms and lotions formulated for dogs and cats suffering from joint or back pain, skin irritations, and wounds. To be absorbed, a topical treatment needs to go directly on the animal's skin.

While the researchers who have studied CBD treatments for dogs and cats have found no significant side effects for the animals, all the experts still advise monitoring pets closely for their reactions. Some animals will become groggy or lethargic from even a small dose of CBD, and they may even experience low blood pressure. Dry mouth is another side effect to watch out for—unlimited access to drinking water is always important, but especially after giving CBD to a pet. If an animal shows any adverse effects from taking CBD, the safe and smart response is to stop the treatment and contact your vet if any problems persist for more than an hour or two after you stop the treatment.

Before giving CBD to any pet, especially those that are taking prescribed medication, be sure to tell your veterinarian about it. This will help ensure that the CBD doesn't counteract or otherwise hamper the effectiveness of the drugs.

Interestingly, CBD may enhance the effects of pharmaceuticals, according to a vet quoted in a 2019 article by *Consumer Reports*. "We do see the strength of pharmaceuticals increase when dogs are taking CBD, so we can often taper down some of those pharmaceuticals," says Casara Andre, D.V.M., founder of Veterinary Cannabis Education and Consulting, a resource for pet owners and veterinarians. "For example, CBD often [amplifies] the effects of antiseizure medications, which is why a lot of times when we combine those with cannabis, we get better control."

PRODUCT CONCERNS

CBD products for pets are not subject to any more regulation than those for humans. That is, manufacturers are not required to test their products on pets or adhere to any quality standards. Pet owners need to read labels and online product information carefully before buying and giving CBD to their dogs and cats. The first step is to look for the seal from the National Animal Supplement Council, which increases the likelihood that a product has been made with safe ingredients in a clean, high-quality environment.

Check for THC content in any CBD pet product and avoid any with more than 0.3 percent THC (the legal limit for hemp-derived products) unless a veterinarian advises otherwise. Independent studies have found more THC in pet products than labels indicate. Evaluations of pet products have also uncovered that some have far less CBD than promised. If the label isn't clear, ask to see a certificate of analysis for any pet product under consideration—it will list the CBD and THC content as well as other ingredients. Reputable brands willingly share this information.

Whether you shop for CBD products for people or pets, online or in stores, you'll notice that oils can be costly. But the AKC's Dr. Klein warns against buying bargain basement products. "The higher the quality and purity, the higher the cost," he says. "You don't want to go for a cheaper option that could have toxic substances such as pesticides, herbicides, or heavy metals. Make sure you buy CBD oil that is free of additives." The best way to be sure of that, he adds, is to buy products made from certified organic hemp.

5

SHOP SMART

HOW TO FIND AND CHOOSE CBD PRODUCTS.

IN THIS CHAPTER

Hemp vs. CBD Oil
Ingestible Products
Topical Products
Quality Matters
Shopping Tips

The explosion of CBD's popularity has many kinds of merchants scrambling to offer it to their customers. CBD products are showing up in retail outlets, from drugstores, supermarkets, and health food shops to fitness clubs, cosmetics counters, and even fast-food restaurants. Countless brands also are promoting CBD products online, each touting unique qualities that distinguish them from all of the others. You'll see a wide array of products infused with CBD, such as vitamin capsules, candies and cookies, energy drinks, lotions for your skin, and soap, as well as oils you can vaporize and inhale.

Your body absorbs CBD oil when you swallow it or dissolve it in your mouth, apply it to your skin, or inhale its vapor. No matter how your body takes in the CBD, it has generally the same effects. But each of the many kinds of products that are used to deliver CBD to your system has distinct differences that impact your experience with it. With such a wide variety of CBD products available, finding the right one for you can seem confusing, but all the options do increase the chances you'll find a product that suits your needs and tastes.

If you're interested in buying CBD, it's a good idea to get familiar with the options, as well as the commonly used terminology and the important attributes to consider. In this chapter, we'll tell you about the pros and cons of each type of product, and explain the factors that can help you find the best quality and value.

HEMP VS. CBD OIL

Hemp is an amazingly versatile plant. Its fiber is used to make textiles for clothing, furniture, and more. Raw or toasted hemp seeds are sold in supermarkets, typically alongside other healthful seeds like flax seed. Hemp oil is used in food, cosmetics, and nutritional supplements and even has industrial applications.

If you're looking for CBD to use for your health, however, you need to understand the critical difference between hemp oil and CBD oil products. Both come from the hemp plant, which refers to strains of the cannabis plant that are low in psychoactive

THC and high in CBD. Hemp oil is made like many other kinds of vegetable oil, such as canola or sunflower oil. That is, it's extracted from the plants' seeds using mechanical pressure. You may see it labeled as "hemp seed" or "hempseed" oil.

Cold-pressed, unrefined hemp seed oil is dark to light green in color, with a nutty flavor. It has a relatively low smoke point (the temperature at which the oil begins to burn, 332°F versus 453°F for vegetable oil), so it is not ideal for cooking. It's more widely used as a finishing oil, in recipes such as pesto, or as a nutritional additive, since it has a rich supply of heart-healthy omega-3 fatty acids.

Refined hemp seed oil is clear and colorless and has little discernible flavor. Many people use it to moisturize their skin and it is also used in body care products, including moisturizing lotions, soaps, and shampoos. Industrial-grade hemp seed oil is used to make lubricants, detergents, paints, inks, fuel, and plastics.

CBD oil also is extracted from the hemp plant, but it comes from the plants' flowers rather than the seeds. The flowers contain the cannabinoids while the seeds have little if any of those compounds. Hemp seed oil is nutritious, but it isn't used for its healing power like CBD oil. Be aware, however, that some CBD products have been found to be mislabeled—perhaps intentionally. These products contain mostly hemp seed oil with just a little of the more expensive CBD oil added. The labels may claim higher "hemp oil" content without clarifying the difference for uninformed consumers.

To further confuse the matter, many good quality CBD

products are labeled as "hemp extract" rather than CBD or CBD oil, because of concerns about the FDA's labeling requirements. When scanning labels, look for terms such as "cannabinoids," "full spectrum," or "broad spectrum" (more on those on page 141) to ensure you are buying CBD and not just hempseed oil.

> **Remember This:** CBD oil (also known as hemp extract) is very different than hemp seed oil, which has little or no cannabinoids and is best used as a food or beauty product.

INGESTIBLE PRODUCTS

Among the many forms of CBD products available these days, you'll find differences in dosage levels, how fast the CBD begins to work, ease of use, and taste. The products fall into two broad categories: ingestibles that you swallow or inhale, and topicals that you apply to your skin. A few basic facts about them, along with a bit of experimentation, will help you figure out which is right for you.

CAPSULES AND SOFTGELS

You are probably familiar with nutritional supplements that you swallow like pills such as vitamins or fish oil. CBD also is available in this form, in many cases blended with other healthful nutrients to help bolster your body's natural defense and healing mechanisms. As you digest the capsule, the CBD is gradually released into your bloodstream and distributed throughout your body. Taking a capsule daily ensures that you have a constant level of cannabinoids available whenever they're needed. Capsules come in a range of concentrations, from 5 milligrams per capsule to 25 milligrams or more, so you can find the exact dose that suits you and ensures you're getting the same dose every time. Swallowing capsules lets you avoid the taste of hemp, which some people find a bit too earthy. The capsules also are free of the sugar found in most edible CBD products.

Used for: Maintaining your body's cannabinoid supply steadily throughout the day.

FIZZY TABLETS

The CBD in tablets that fizz when plopped in water (like Alka-Seltzer) is more quickly absorbed than capsules, gels, or gummies that must go through digestion before entering the bloodstream. Be aware, however, that CBD oil is not water-soluble, so these kinds of effervescent tablets are most often made with CBD isolate, a crystalline form of CBD from which terpenes, flavonoids, and many other beneficial compounds that are found in the oil have been stripped. (More on CBD isolate on page 142.)

Used for: Effervescent tablets are a fast-working option that may help calm an attack of pain, anxiety, or stress.

TINCTURE OR DROPS

CBD tincture (commonly referred to as CBD drops) is CBD oil blended with pure alcohol and, frequently, another plant-based oil, such as coconut or sesame, to make it easier for you to use. You can choose from a variety of concentrations, ranging from

500 milligrams of CBD per bottle to 1,500 milligrams and more—higher concentrations deliver more CBD per drop. The "green tea" herbal flavor becomes more pronounced as you go from lower to higher concentrations. With CBD tinctures, you calibrate the dosage by adjusting the number of drops you take, which can be inexact if you're not vigilant.

Squirting a few drops under your tongue is the most popular way to use tinctures. Hold it there for 30 seconds before swallowing so that the CBD is absorbed through the mucous membrane at the bottom of your mouth. Used this way, the CBD can begin to work in as little as 10 minutes—faster than swallowing it. Concentrations vary from one product to another, so check labels to determine how much CBD is in each drop.

Many CBD users add a few drops of tincture to smoothies, fresh juice, or other food and drinks to disguise the flavor or to take CBD as part of their healthy diet. CBD tincture ingested this way goes through your digestive process and takes 30 minutes or more to enter your bloodstream.

Used for: Those seeking quick relief from insomnia, anxiety, or other acute conditions often rely on the fast absorption of CBD drops.

SUBLINGUAL STRIPS

Like the breath fresheners many people use, CBD oil is blended with flavorings like mint and made into clear "filmy" strips that dissolve quickly in your mouth. The CBD is absorbed through the mucous membranes in your palate. Sublingual strips come in a range of doses for you to choose from, starting as low as 5 milligrams. They are typically low in calories and sugar-free. The mint flavoring freshens your breath and helps mute the taste and aroma of CBD. The strips come in handy packs that let you slip one in your mouth whenever you're ready for a dose of CBD.

Used for: Situations when you want a fast dose of CBD and you want to remain discreet.

ORAL OR NASAL SPRAYS

A spritz of atomized oil in your mouth or nose can give a swiftly absorbed dose of 1 to 3 milligrams of CBD. The pump bottle sprays directly into the permeable mucus membranes—easy to do just about anywhere. When using oral CBD, try to get the spray under your tongue or on your cheeks where it can dissolve before you swallow. Oral sprays come in flavors like vanilla and peppermint, leaving you with a pleasant taste in your mouth. Be sure to thoroughly shake the bottle each time you pump, because CBD oil may separate from the water in the bottle and cling to the sides.

Used for: When you need a small dose of CBD quickly.

SWEETS

Gummy bears, chocolate bars, hard candy, chewing gum, cookies, and other "edibles" might be the most palatable way to ingest CBD, though the earthy flavor of CBD oil is typically masked by excess sugar or other sweeteners. Edibles are often the choice for people who give CBD to children or senior citizens because they are so readily taken. (Note: Discuss with your family doctor before giving CBD to children or older people.) Edibles make it easy to regulate exactly how much of a dose you get. Like with any product you swallow, it takes about a half hour for the CBD to get into your bloodstream. (Chewing gum is an exception—you don't swallow it and it may begin working sooner since some of the CBD is absorbed through the mucus membranes in your mouth.) Wrapped candies should stay potent for weeks if they're kept in a cool, dry location. Baked foods, such as brownies and cookies, should be stored in the refrigerator to keep the CBD oil fresh for a few weeks.

Used for: People who find the taste of CBD oil unpleasant.

FUNCTIONAL FOODS

Gyms, health-food stores, drugstores, and supermarkets carry performance-boosting energy bars and sports drinks enhanced with CBD. They're promoted as an aid to speed recovery from hard workouts. A former NFL star, Terrell Davis, has launched a line of CBD-infused sports drinks called Defy. H20 Balance, OKI, and Aethics are other brands offering products for pre- and postworkout. You may also find CBD "shots," blended with herbal stimulants and sold in individual bottles and cans much like quick-hit energy drinks. Dosages vary in these products from 5 to 20 milligrams.

Used for: Getting a dose of CBD to relieve soreness and aches after demanding exercise.

DAILY DIET

When a nutritional supplement is offered as an additive to food and drink in trendy restaurants and cafes, it may have reached a peak of cultural awareness. That's happening with CBD. An Indian restaurant in New York City, for instance, put CBD-infused ghee (clarified butter) on its menu. (The city has since banned using CBD as a food additive.) At one Carl's Jr. fast-food location, there was a special promotion that included a hamburger with CBD added to the meat. Several brewing companies offer CBD-infused beer and distillers are making vodka, tequila, and other liquors with the compound. You can find coffee and tea products containing CBD, or you can pick up CBD honey sticks or straws to dissolve in any drink. A Pennsylvania company is marketing gelato that comes with a dose of CBD. Some retailers offer coffee, tea, cocktails, smoothies, and other healthy drinks with added CBD on the list of options a customer can request.

The trend is now attracting major food industry corporations, too. Coca-Cola and Molson Coors Brewing, for instance, are developing CBD products, according to media reports.

The FDA, however, announced in December 2018, a prohibition against introducing "food containing added CBD or THC into interstate commerce. This is because CBD and THC are active ingredients in FDA-approved drugs and were the subject of substantial clinical investigations before they were marketed as foods or dietary supplements. Under the Food, Drug and Cosmetics Act, it is illegal to introduce drug ingredients like these into the food supply," said Scott Gottlieb, M.D., administrator of the

FDA. Some states and cities across the country are banning the sale of food and drink with added CBD.

Used for: Sampling CBD in a familiar form.

VAPE OIL

E-cigarettes were invented to give smokers a dose of nicotine without the harmful effects of inhaling burning tobacco leaves. Instead, they inhale the vapor from heated oil. This same technology is used to deliver a dose of CBD (or THC or both). Vape (short for vaporizer) pens or tanks contain a small cartridge with the oil, which is heated by a coil warmed by battery power. The oil vaporizes and the user inhales the steam. Vaporized CBD tends to enter the bloodstream faster than in any other form—in as quickly as 30 seconds or less, according to Mitch Earleywine, Ph.D., a professor of psychology at the State University of New York, Albany, in an article published by *Consumer Reports* in 2018.

Managing your dosage can be challenging when you vape. The concentration of CBD (or THC) in the oil varies widely from one brand to the next. And how hard and how long you inhale has a direct impact on how much of the cannabinoids you ingest. Start with a single inhale, then wait a few minutes and see whether there is an effect. If not, try another. With experience, regular vape users learn to calibrate the dosage for their needs. By the way, avoid holding your breath after inhaling, because that can irritate your lungs and does not increase the amount of CBD you absorb.

A solvent called propylene glycol is used in e-cigarettes

containing nicotine and in CBD vape oils. (The solvent is often used in asthma inhalers, too.) It keeps the oil and any added flavorings blended together and in liquid form, and it helps "smoke clouds" to form when you inhale the vapors. At high temperatures, propylene glycol can degrade into formaldehyde, a chemical that can irritate your nose and eyes and could increase your risk of asthma and cancer.

Bear in mind that vape makers are required to inform the FDA about their products, but there is no public disclosure. Companies can tell customers as much or as little as they want. Also, beware of exceptionally low-priced vaping oils—some have been found to contain diethylene glycol, an industrial solvent that is poisonous. Checking labels and certificates of analysis is especially crucial for vaping oils.

The practice of vaping itself has come under scrutiny by public health officials. Reports of illnesses and even deaths are increasing among people who are heavy vapers of nicotine- or cannabis-based oils. While most experts believe that vaping is less harmful than smoking, it is not without risks. Research is just beginning into the long-term effects of vaping and the ingredients used in the oils. You can avoid the risks by choosing other forms of CBD.

Used for: Those seeking quick relief for anxiety, seizures, and other acute conditions.

DAB, WAX, AND OTHER CONCENTRATES

CBD oil (with or without THC) can be refined and concentrated into solids of various kinds, most commonly referred to as "dab," "wax," or "shatter." They are each slightly different, but all have a high concentration of cannabinoids, so you get a strong dose quickly from inhaling the vapor. The concentrates are placed in a "rig" or water pipe that looks similar to the "bongs" used to smoke marijuana. When heated, the concentrates vaporize and the steam is inhaled to ingest the CBD.

These products are not as widely available as other forms of CBD, so many users make them on their own from fresh cannabis flowers. This process tends to be complicated and can be costly because a substantial amount of cannabis is needed to produce the concentrates.

Used for: Experienced CBD and cannabis users who want a strong, immediate dose of CBD, typically for acute pain or anxiety.

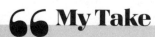
My Take

I recently started using a CBD infused facial serum that I love. I've had some areas of redness on my face as well as fine lines. I don't really have what one would call wrinkles. I've been using it for 2 weeks. The redness is fading and my face feels really relaxed after applying it. I have seen a decrease in the fine lines around my mouth. I will continue to purchase this product.
—**Deb Barger, Athens, Alabama**

TOPICAL PRODUCTS

CBD can be absorbed through your skin so many people with aches and pains or skin conditions use topical products to relieve their symptoms.

LOTIONS, CREAMS, AND BALMS

CBD oil is blended with fats such as coconut oil or beeswax to make creams, lotions, and balms that users apply right where they want the CBD to work. Users typically report that they begin feeling the effects 30 to 45 minutes after the application and for up to three hours after that.

Topical products come in various forms and strengths. Many are like moisturizing lotions that can be spread over arms, legs, necks, and shoulders or rubbed into pain joints. Balms, like many over-the-counter pain-relief rubs, are thicker than the creams and often come with other well-known soothing ingredients such as menthol. Because of their consistency, balms work well for massaging into targeted spots.

Topical CBD applications are most popular for treating chronic pain of the joints and other specific spots on the body and for dealing with skin conditions, such as acne and eczema.

Used for: Treating pain "hot spots" or skin conditions caused by inflammation.

COSMETICS

Many cosmetics brands take advantage of the latest trends in health and wellness to keep their products up-to-date. So, no surprise, you can now find moisturizers, antiaging creams, lip gloss, mascara, skin scrubs, specialty soaps, blemish treatments, shampoo and other hair care products, and even toothpaste formulated with CBD oil. Unlike lotions, creams, and balms that are designed to treat specific hot spots on your body, CBD cosmetics have low doses, so they would only contribute to maintaining your body's overall levels of CBD rather than treating a particular condition. There's no research showing that the kind of minute amounts of CBD found in cosmetics have any benefit.

Cosmetics and other topicals are governed by different FDA regulations than food and drink. Cannabis-derived ingredients are permitted in products that are not consumed. But as with all CBD products, the FDA prohibits claims about healing specific conditions in the marketing of these products.

Used for: Looking good while you're feeling good.

BATH BOMBS AND SALTS

Many people, from professional athletes and weekend warriors to folks looking for a little stress relief, enjoy soaking in warm water to soothe their sore muscles and relax their minds. They can try to enhance the experience by adding bath salts and bombs blended with CBD. The bath products are meant to act as a gentle anti-inflammatory for the whole body. The formulas typically include essential oils from other medicinal herbs, such as lavender, chamomile, and arnica, which have long been used to treat common aches and pains and stress. People with chronic foot pain also use CBD bath salts for soaking their feet.

Bath products come with higher doses of CBD—250 milligrams or more—than you generally find in products you ingest. That's because your whole body is absorbing the compound rather than just your digestive system. Customers reviewing a CBD bath product online noted that it was effective at reducing the swelling and itching that result from bug bites and it soothed inflamed and scaly skin.

Used for: Adding extra anti-inflammatory relief to a soothing hot bath.

SKIN PATCHES

"Transdermal" patches are widely used to deliver pain relievers and other medications, hormones, and nicotine at a steady rate over a long period of time. The sticky patch is applied to the skin and the active ingredients are gradually absorbed and distributed throughout the body. CBD patches that work the same way are now on the market.

A skin patch offers benefits that appeal to certain groups of users. Those who suffer from chronic aches and pains throughout their bodies—such as fibromyalgia patients—can get a constant, moderate supply of CBD from a skin patch. Cancer patients use CBD patches to help with their symptoms, including loss of appetite. Anyone who finds other forms of CBD products unpalatable might consider using a skin patch.

Skin patches are available with doses ranging from 5 to 50 milligrams. Typically, the CBD is released over a 12-hour period. Because the patch delivers a consistent dose, there's almost no chance of overuse. If you choose to try a CBD patch, be sure to apply it to clean, dry, and unbroken skin—open wounds or inflamed skin may be irritated by the patch and its ingredients.

Used for: People who want to maintain consistent levels of CBD for relief from constant pain and other symptoms.

> **Remember This:** As you consider CBD products for yourself, take note of how they differ in absorption rate, their application to specific conditions, and their palatability.

QUALITY MATTERS

The popularity of CBD has enticed many brands to introduce the wide range of products covered in the preceding section. But just as these CBD delivery methods vary greatly, so does that quality and quantity of the CBD they contain. In this section you'll find out what the different attributes mean and what to look for when shopping for products you want to use.

Before you think about making a purchase, bear in mind that neither the FDA nor any other government agency regulates the contents of CBD products. The government does prohibit unsubstantiated health claims for CBD, just like it would for any other supplement or herbal remedy, but all of the responsibility for testing and validating the products lies with the brands that sell them.

And many of the brands are actively misleading consumers. In 2017, a team from the University of Pennsylvania School of Medicine published the results of their study of CBD products in the *Journal of the American Medical Association (JAMA).* The research team, led by Marcel Bonn-Miller, Ph.D., an adjunct assistant professor of psychology in Psychiatry, purchased and analyzed 84 products from 31 different companies and found that more than 42 percent of products were underlabeled, meaning that the product contained a higher concentration of

CBD than indicated. Another 26 percent of products purchased were overlabeled, meaning the product contained a lower concentration of CBD than indicated. Only 30 percent of CBD products purchased contained an actual CBD content that was within 10 percent of the amount listed on the product label. The researchers noted that some of the CBD products they analyzed also contained a significant amount of THC—the chemical compound in cannabis responsible for making a person feel intoxicated.

UNDERSTANDING EXTRACTION

CBD processors use one of a few different methods for extracting the cannabinoid from the plant. Which method used has a meaningful impact on the other compounds that come with it, and it affects the quality, costs, and best uses for the final product. The methods explained here are often mentioned in product information, so understanding them can help you make more informed choices in a confusing marketplace.

Solvent. Ethanol or another potent form of alcohol acts as a solvent, pulling the CBD from the plants. The hemp flowers soak in the ethanol, then the excess liquid is poured off. The remainder is heated and distilled to concentrate it. While "solvent" sounds like a toxic substance, ethanol is listed by the FDA as "generally regarded as safe," and it is commonly used as a food preservative and additive found in many products at the grocery store

The heat from the distillation process also can burn off other desirable compounds that come with the CBD, such as terpenes and flavonoids that may enhance the effectiveness of the CBD. Extraction by solvent is a common choice for small operations and for producers of vaping oils, because the results are easy to work with. This is the simplest method of extraction, requires minimal skill, and is least costly in terms of equipment and power. But if not done properly, unwanted residues from the solvents can remain in the oil. Premium brands typically use the next method, CO_2 extraction.

Carbon dioxide. CO_2 extraction is a more complex process involving several steps. Carbon dioxide is put under high pressure and kept at extremely low temperatures until it becomes what's known to scientists as "supercritical," meaning it shares properties with both gas and liquid. As the supercritical CO_2 is pushed through cannabis flowers, it dissolves the CBD and other compounds from the plant matter.

Carbon dioxide extraction requires elaborate equipment and expensive supplies. And it takes full attention to the details. Many producers automate some of the steps, which helps ensure consistency in the end product. Since no chemicals other than CO_2 are used in this process, there are no residues left behind. The cold temperatures used in CO_2 extraction help to preserve terpenes and other heat-sensitive compounds. This method is the most efficient at extracting the available CBD. Products made with CBD oil extracted with CO_2 (which you'll see on their labels) may be more costly than those extracted with solvents, but they also are likely to be the safest to use and to come with the full complement of beneficial ingredients.

Hydrocarbons. CBD products such as wax, dab, or shatter

are thick concentrates that are potent and fast-acting. They are heated and the vapors they emit are inhaled. Hydrocarbon solvents—typically butane, hexane, propane, or a combination—are used to extract the CBD from the cannabis flowers. This process works very well at capturing the cannabinoids and terpenes without chlorophyll and other undesirable compounds. The result is thick, tree-like sap.

While some manufacturers use hydrocarbons because this method is fast and inexpensive, many THC aficionados are making their own concentrates at home with it. It can be risky. Hydrocarbons are highly flammable and toxic. Any residue left in the extract might be harmful to your health. For those reasons, hydrocarbon extraction is best left to people with experience and proper equipment.

Oil or butter. You can make CBD oil in your own kitchen, in a process just like people have long used to extract THC from marijuana to add to brownies and other edibles. You don't even need elaborate equipment—just a baking sheet, saucepan, and ordinary olive (or coconut) oil or butter.

You start by baking 1 cup of cannabis flowers on a tray in the oven at a low temperature (245°F) for 30 to 40 minutes. Gently shake the tray every 10 minutes to be sure the flowers heat through uniformly. This process is called "decarboxylation," or "decarbing," and it is necessary to activate the CBD. (More on that process in the next section.)

When the flowers are thoroughly dried, you want to grind them by hand (an old coffee grinder is handy for this). After the cannabis is coarsely ground, you are ready to add 1 cup of water and 1 cup of oil or butter to a saucepan. Simmer at a low temperature (between 160° and 200°F), then pour the cannabis into the pot as the butter melts. Maintain the simmer at the low heat for two to three hours, stirring occasionally. The mixture should never come to a full boil, as the heat can cook off the CBD.

Once the liquid starts to thicken into melted oil or butter, turn off the heat and let it cool. Place a funnel on top of a jar and line it with cheesecloth. Pour the oil or butter over the cheese-cloth funnel and allow it to strain freely. (Tip: Squeezing the cheesecloth may push more bad-tasting plant material through so avoid doing that). Store the CBD butter or oil in the refrigerator where it should stay effective for three to four weeks.

This process can be challenging to do on your own, but DIY types may find it rewarding. If you decide to try it, keep in mind that it is the least efficient way to get CBD oil. You need a cup of CBD-rich hemp flowers to make a cup of oil.

Decarboxylation. This is a complex-sounding term that is more relevant to CBD producers than consumers. You may notice, however, that many brands include this term in their product descriptions. A brief explanation will help you under-stand why it shows up in consumer information and why products that do not go through this process may not be effective.

Cannabis flowers don't actually contain CBD (or even THC). Rather, they have what are called raw acid precursors, which are abbreviated as CBDA (or THCA). You can think of them like the beta-carotene in foods—it is not a nutrient your body uses directly, but in your digestive process the nutrient is converted into vitamin A, which does nourish you. When a low-temperature process—such as CO2 extraction—is used to produce CBD, the compound must be activated to transform CBDA into CBD. Applying heat changes the molecules so that the acid is released and the CBD remains. That process is decarboxylation.

That said, researchers are studying how these "raw" molecules interact differently with our body's endocannabinoid systems and whether they may offer some benefits that CBD does not. These inquiries are in their early stages, so you still want to be sure that the CBD products you consider buying have gone through the "decarb" process.

> **Remember This:** CBD extracted using the CO2 method will be free of residues from the solvents and other chemicals used in other methods.

FULL, BROAD, OR ISOLATE

Three other terms describing the quality of the CBD oil in products show up on many labels and descriptions. Full spectrum, broad spectrum, and isolate refer to the contents of CBD oil besides the CBD itself.

Full spectrum. The flowers of the hemp plant contain a wide range of compounds besides CBD. These include terpenes, essential oils, fatty acids, flavonoids, chlorophyll, and other cannabinoids besides CBD. And the strains of cannabis that are classified as "hemp" because they are not psychoactive may have trace amounts of THC (though not enough to make you feel intoxicated). Full-spectrum CBD oil comes with all of those other compounds. Many experts and consumers believe that these elements work together to magnify the therapeutic benefits of CBD alone. You will hear this referred to as the "entourage effect" (see page 69). Products made with full-spectrum CBD oil typically have the distinct flavor of hemp, which has been likened to that of green or herbal tea.

Broad spectrum. Some brands offer products made with broad-spectrum CBD oil, which has nearly all of the same compounds found in full-spectrum products. That means broad-spectrum products may still deliver the benefits of the entourage effect. And broad-spectrum CBD oil may taste "grassy," just as full spectrum does.

Broad-spectrum CBD oil, however, has gone through an extra step in processing to remove even the most miniscule traces of THC. For people who are subject to drug testing and those who are extremely sensitive to THC intoxication, broad-spectrum CBD oil is a much safer choice than full spectrum.

Isolate. When CBD is purified—often into a crystalline powder form rather than in an oil—it is transformed into an "isolate." It contains up to 99.9 percent CBD and no other compounds such as THC, terpenes, flavonoids, or other nutrients. There is no "entourage effect" with isolates. They have little or no taste or aroma. Isolates are often used in products because they are the least expensive to make and use, the contents are consistent and predictable, and the powder blends well with other ingredients, since they do not affect the flavor. If you want to make your own CBD edibles such as baked goods or use CBD in smoothies or similar drinks, isolates make it easy for you. Products made with isolates are the safest choice for anyone who is subject to testing for THC.

> **Remember This:** "Full-spectrum" CBD products may have trace amounts of THC, though still below the legal limit. If you want to avoid THC altogether, choose products made with "broad-spectrum" CBD or isolates.

CBD PLUS THC

Let's begin here with a quick review: THC is the intoxicant in marijuana and possession of it in any form is illegal under federal law. More than 30 states have legalized medicinal THC, and 11 of them permit any adult to use it. On the other hand, CBD products are not intoxicating, and, while federal law about them is currently unclear, there is widespread agreement that consumers are not at legal risk for buying or using them (see page 18 for more details). Remember that CBD and THC both come from the flower buds of the same plant species, cannabis. Strains high in THC are classified as "marijuana," while those with less than 0.3 percent THC are legally known as "hemp."

Cannabis breeders—amateurs and pros—are an exceptionally enterprising group of people. For many years, they worked to develop varieties that had higher and higher levels of THC, because that's what marijuana customers wanted. But as buzz about the benefits of CBD has grown recently, they've been hybridizing varieties with a balance of both cannabinoids.

The extracts from these plants have more equal (though not exactly) concentrations of THC and CBD. For many people, THC enhances the "entourage effect" and is better able to relieve their symptoms than CBD alone.

You can get these "two-way" products only in states where THC use is permitted. And many brands in the fast-growing THC marketplace are adding more of the balanced products to their lines because of the popularity of CBD. Responsible vendors disclose the THC and CBD content in their products on labels or sites, so you can make an informed choice.

> **Remember This:** For many people, CBD products are even more effective when they include THC, but these products are not legal everywhere.

ADDITIVE AWARENESS

CBD extracted from hemp is just one component of nearly all products with CBD on the label. The extract is blended with other ingredients to make it palatable or useful. In topical products, the other components typically are other kinds of oil, such as coconut or olive, as well as herbs with a long history in folk medicine, such as lavender, eucalyptus, and chamomile. Candy and other edible items include sweeteners and flavorings. The best quality products are made without artificial sweeteners, colors, or flavors.

Tinctures are made by mixing the CBD with pure alcohol and other food-grade oils, such as MCT (medium-chain triglycerides), which is extracted from coconut oil. In the rush to get CBD products on the market, some manufacturers bulk up their products with cheaper hemp seed oil or other inert fillers.

Additives are of greatest concern when buying products for vaping. Manufacturers of these often blend the CBD oil with propylene glycol (PG) to help the CBD heat up evenly and produce substantial amounts of vapor. (PG is also regularly included in nicotine-infused liquids that are used in e-cigarettes.) PG is classified by the FDA as "generally recognized as safe" and is approved for ingestion as a food additive. It has not, however, been safety tested by the FDA for inhalation when heated. While no problems have been attributed directly to inhalation of PG, you will be safer choosing products made with vegetable glycerin instead.

Like nicotine oils for e-cigarettes, CBD vape products are often flavored to make them more appealing to consumer tastes. These flavoring agents are approved by the FDA for ingestion and topical application, but not for inhalation. Diacetyl is a compound added to vape oil cartridges to simulate various buttery flavors, ranging from cream to vanilla and caramel. Diacetyl has been linked to respiratory illness in several studies.

In recent years, synthetic cannabinoids often marketed as "K2" or "Spice" have attracted consumers seeking a legal high that is akin to marijuana. The most prevalent, known to scientists as 5F-ADB, has been linked to damaging overdoses and even deaths. In 2018, a team of researchers at Virginia Commonwealth University analyzed seven products labeled as CBD that contained 5F-ADB and Dextromethorphan (DMX), an ingredient in cough medicine that has a history of recreational abuse and associated health problems. To prevent exposure to these potentially dangerous chemicals, look at the ingredient labels on any vaping product you are considering buying—be wary of any brand that won't share the contents of its products.

DOSAGE DIFFERENCES

Let's begin by making clear that except for the FDA-approved epilepsy medication made with CBD, no research has firmly established the ideal dosages to get the full benefits of the cannabinoid. (For more on that, go to page 89.) To further complicate the matter, CBD products come in a wide range of dosages, and the information that brands provide about the right amount for you can be unsubstantiated and misleading.

If you plan on ingesting CBD, most experts and experienced users recommend starting with small amounts and waiting a week before gradually increasing the dosage as you observe how you feel and find your tolerance level. Products with controlled dosages, such as capsules, candy, and skin patches, make it easier for you to manage your intake than drops or vaping. When you apply CBD lotion or balm to your skin, you can take a higher dosage without concerns about overdoing it.

LABEL LANGUAGE

The FDA requires a few specific pieces of information on the labels of products classified as either food or dietary supplement, categories that include most types of CBD products.

Reading and understanding that information can help you find the best choices for you.

Products with CBD that are intended to be food, such as candy bars or sports drinks, must have nutrition facts (calories, protein, fats, vitamins, and minerals) on their labels. Food labels also must list ingredients. Use of the word "hemp" in the product descriptions on the front of packages can be confusing. Check the ingredient list to be sure it includes CBD oil, or cannabis or hemp extract, not hemp seeds or hemp seed oil.

Capsules and tablets, drops, gummies and other sweets, and even energy bars and other functional foods are categorized as dietary supplements. The fronts of these packages must specify the net weight (volume of the container for liquids) or the count (number of capsules or tablets contained in the bottle). On the back, you'll find a Supplement Facts panel that lists the amount (in milligrams) of hemp extract, CBD oil, or isolate per serving.

To make an informed purchase, you need to take note of the total amount of CBD in each product and the recommended amount per dose. A 30-milliliter bottle of tincture, for instance, may come with 500 milligrams of CBD. If a 150-pound person takes about 35 milligrams per day (as suggested on page 89), the bottle of tincture has approximately 14 doses. A 300 milligram bottle of gummy bears that are 5 milligrams each amounts to about eight or nine doses. Keep that in mind as you assess the value of products you are considering.

One more helpful bit of information can be gleaned from product labels: Where was the hemp grown and processed?

Until 2018, growing hemp was illegal in the United States and so American brands had to source their raw material from overseas, including Europe where it has been legal to raise it. Growers in Western European countries and the United States are subject to regulations governing the types and amounts of agricultural pesticides, fungicides, and other chemicals that can be used on any crop—that's none if the crops are certified organic. But the fast-growing demand for CBD products has attracted growers in parts of the world where regulation is lax or nonexistent. Your safest bet is to be wary of any brand that doesn't tell the origins of its hemp on its labels or website.

The FDA maintains strict standards for health claims on the labels of dietary supplements. It prohibits statements that directly link the product or any of its components to treatments for specific conditions—labels can't say "reduces your risk of cancer" or "relieves arthritis pain" unless that's been proven and accepted by the agency. Dietary supplements can make what the FDA calls "structure/function claims," that describe how the key nutrient or ingredient affects the normal structure or function of the human body. For example, "cannabinoids play a role in your body's pain management system." These regulations explain why reputable CBD products aren't labeled as treatments for exact health disorders.

LAB TESTING

How can you trust what's in the CBD product you are buying? The FDA doesn't test the products, and its regulations are similar to those imposed on makers of any dietary supplement: Ingredient lists must be truthful, and labels, ads, or other consumer information cannot make unapproved health claims. Still, every reputable CBD brand submits their products to independent laboratory testing and will share the certificate of analysis either online or, upon request, via email. The certificate (often referred to as the COA) will tell you the product's CBD and THC levels and what other compounds are present, including both desirable ones like terpenes as well as unwanted contaminants.

Check the certificate to see if the lab meets "ISO 17025" standards, which ensure the credibility of its results. This designation denotes that the lab adheres to high scientific standards. The most trustworthy labs also employ testing methods validated by one of three respected national standard-setting organizations: the Association of Official Agricultural Chemists (aoac.org), American Herbal Pharmacopoeia (herbal-ahp.org), and US Pharmacopeia (usp.org).

State legislators in Indiana and Utah wanted to prevent the sale of products labeled as CBD that have more than negligible amounts of THC—they feared brands would do this to skirt the restrictions on marijuana sales. So those states have passed a strict labeling law requiring that every CBD product sold in the state come with a QR code. The QR codes must direct consumers to detailed information about each CBD product, including its batch number, expiration date, ingredients, and an independent lab analysis.

Remember This: Every reputable brand of CBD products will let you see its certificate of analysis (COA), a lab report on its contents.

WHY ORGANIC

You may be familiar with the reasons for buying organic food and other products. They are raised and processed without pesticides or fungicides, synthetic fertilizers, or genetically modified organisms (often referred to as GMOs). These practices and many others by organic farmers help protect the environment and yield food that is cleaner and safer for people.

When it comes to CBD products, it may be even more important to choose the organic option. Cannabis acts as a "bio-accumulator," meaning that the plant draws heavy metals, toxic chemicals, and other contaminants out of the soil. This attribute makes the plants useful for cleaning up areas where industrial waste has been dumped. (It's been reported that hemp was planted at the site of the 1988 Chernobyl nuclear reactor disaster for this purpose.)

Of course, you don't want CBD from plants grown in toxic waste, but hemp grown with pesticides, herbicides, and fungicides will come with residues from those chemicals. There may be only a few parts per billion on each plant, but the CBD extraction process concentrates the compounds in the flowers. To avoid getting a dose of contaminants with your CBD, go with products made with certified organic hemp, which is grown without agricultural chemicals.

SHOPPING TIPS

Even after you've finished wading through all of the product options available, you still have to decide where to buy. You see lots of choices in retail stores and online. In this section, we'll help you to zero in on sources that meet your expectations.

ABOUT THE PRICE

We know you've noticed. The prices on CBD products can be steep. You aren't likely to find anything but "trial" packs of almost any type of product that costs less than $40. As the concentration of CBD increases, the prices can climb quickly past $100 for a month's supply. At 10 cents per milligram, pure CBD oil would cost $2,835 an ounce—the kind of price paid for precious metals.

That is substantially more than aspirin, vitamins, or other dietary supplements. Many willingly pay these prices because the products bring them relief. But you may be asking why must CBD cost so much. The simple rules of supply and demand are the primary reason. CBD is extracted from the flowers of the hemp plant, which must be raised vigilantly to ensure that it produces oil-rich buds instead of seeds. And it takes a lot of those flowers to make CBD oil. Experienced growers estimate that each plant bears about 1 pound of flowers and about an acre of land can yield up to 2,500 plants. Depending on the strain, a pound of flowers produces 40 to 50 milligrams of CBD oil.

With federal restrictions on growing hemp in the United States, the supply of plants for processing into CBD has been limited. In states that have legalized marijuana production and Kentucky (which has incentivized its tobacco farmers to convert to hemp), the existing acreage devoted to growing cannabis is increasing fast. And farmers in states where raising hemp has been prohibited are now planting the crop to take advantage of the lucrative returns it can earn—more than any of the common commodity crops, such as corn or soybeans. In those places, the 2019 growing season was the first time farmers have been able to plant it. Even though so many growers are ramping up quickly, demand for CBD products is rising faster. For now, that's keeping prices high.

Processing hemp to make CBD is also newly legal in the United States, so the number and capacity of operations able to extract the oil is small, though it is now growing rapidly. When the supply of raw material (cannabis plants) and efficiencies in processing catch up to the demand for CBD products, prices are likely to come down.

In the meantime, you can find good deals with smart shopping. Many brands offer discounts to first-time buyers and veterans, who often treat chronic pain and/or PTSD with CBD products. Some brands offer price breaks and other kinds of assistance to low-income customers.

Doing a price comparison of the wide variety of CBD products can be confusing. A smart way to start is to determine the cost per milligram you're paying. You'll find some products costing as little as 5 cents per milligram, others at 20 cents or more. As you do the comparison, you may find that the product with the lowest retail price has a higher cost per milligram than a more expensive product.

We won't call this a hard and fast rule, but in our survey of a wide variety of brands and products, capsules and tablets generally have the lowest cost per milligram with vaping oils and tinctures the next most cost-effective. Topicals and cosmetics typically come with the highest price tags, both overall and on a per-milligram-of-CBD basis—that may be attributed to the costs of other ingredients and the prices of comparable products that don't contain CBD.

The high costs can tempt you to look for bargain basement products. But you should be wary of any item that costs dramatically less than comparable products. Keep in mind that the CBD market is new, growing fast, and largely unregulated. In a hot market with little oversight, unscrupulous vendors are finding ways to shortcut or skimp on the active ingredients. Some use imported hemp extract that may have very little CBD from countries such as China, where farmers and processors aren't subject to any regulations. A good rule to remember is that you get what you pay for—if a product is unbelievably cheap, you should question its trustworthiness.

> **Remember This:** Products priced well below the market are likely to be very low in CBD or even have nontherapeutic hemp seed oil.

BETTER BRANDS

There are dozens of brands selling CBD products and more entering the marketplace every day. There are no specific endorsements here, but with a little information you can identify good quality CBD products and reputable brands yourself.

An industry group, the US Hemp Authority (USHA), has developed a certification program for hemp products to set "high standards, best practices and self-regulation, giving confidence to consumers and law enforcement that hemp products are safe and legal." The USHA's list of standards is long and technical, but it addresses the whole process of producing CBD, from hemp growing, extraction, sampling and testing, quality control, and labeling. Throughout, the emphasis is on providing consumers with transparent and credible information.

To be certified, brands must adhere to stringent standards for self-regulation and pass a third-party audit. Those that are approved can use a certified seal on their packaging and promotional materials. Launched in 2019, this program has already enrolled more than 60 hemp brands. You can find them all listed on the USHA website (ushempauthority.org).

When considering buying products from any brand, look for those that make it easy for you to review their certificate of analysis, are clear and thorough in their ingredients lists, and provide details about the source and place of origin for the hemp used to produce it. Brands sold in retail outlets such as supermarkets and drug stores have been vetted by the store's buyers—a layer of approval that online-only products don't face.

A few brands are already emerging as market leaders with reputable products. To help you get started on choosing a brand to buy, a few of them are listed here.

Bluebird Botanicals was an early entrant into the CBD

market, and it has remained a popular brand of oils, creams, capsules, vape oil, isolates, and products formulated for pets. Bluebird's "Lot/Batch Numbering System" lets you see the certificate of analysis for the exact container of the product you buy. The products are available through health-care providers and retail stores as well as online. The company is USHA certified. Learn more at bluebirdbotanicals.com.

CV Sciences is developing prescription pharmaceuticals made with hemp extract as well as over-the-counter consumer products. Under its PlusCBDoil brand, you can find capsules and soft gels, tincture and oral spray, topical balm and roll-on, and gummies. They are distributed nationally in health food stores, health-care providers' offices, and online. The company is USHA certified. Learn more at pluscbdoil.com.

CW Hemp is the company behind Charlotte's Web tinctures, capsules, gummies, and pet products. They're made with the extract of a high-CBD strain of hemp called "Charlotte's Web." CW Hemp has been certified by the USHA. The products are in retail outlets nationwide and are available online. Learn more at charlottesweb.com.

Lazarus Naturals offers scented balms, flavored oils (both full spectrum and isolates), and capsules. All of its products are made with only vegan ingredients. The hemp used is grown in central Oregon, but the products are available in natural health stores and other retail outlets nationwide and online. Learn more at lazarusnaturals.com.

Medterra products, including capsules, creams, oil, and pet items, are guaranteed to be THC-free. Some of its capsule and gel formulations feature CBD blended with other natural healing ingredients, such as melatonin and valerian root. The pet oils come in beef and chicken flavors. Medterra is USHA certified. Its products are available in natural health stores and similar retailers nationwide and online. Learn more at medterracbd.com.

66 My Take

I am a retired family physician. I have never used marijuana. However, for the past 10 years I had had several major medical problems, including fibromyalgia and general malaise. Because of all of the positive articles and press about CBD oil, and after speaking with my pharmacist and physician, I decided to try it in hopes that it would help.

But I also have MCS, multiple chemical sensitivity, and have sensitivity to wood products. When I bought a CBD oil tincture, I sniffed it first and was a bit concerned, but proceeded to try it because I was hopeful to have positive results. The recommended starting dose is 20 drops or 10 milligrams. I put only 3 drops or 1.5 milligrams in my mouth. I was terribly wrong! The CBD tincture tasted like 3-in-1 oil mixed with pine resin and turpentine. My mouth stung. I should have rinsed it out immediately, but I did not. Instead I swallowed. Major Mistake!

All night I was hot and flushed and felt "antsy"—absolutely no rest! In the morning I continued to feel ill. That afternoon I began getting sicker. I continued to smell and taste the CBD oil for nearly 36 hours! I have no idea what would have happened to me if I had taken the full recommended starting dose. So, CBD oil is not a panacea . . . and is definitely not for individuals who are chemically sensitive or have sensitivities to wood products.

—Kathleen Beine, M.D., Kingsport, Tennessee

99

CBD STRAINS

Back in the days when marijuana was sold only on the black market, baggies of pot often came with names like "Panama Red," "Columbian Gold," and "Maui Wowie." Those were purportedly the strains of cannabis from which the marijuana was harvested, and the names were meant to get customers excited about the potency and other desirable qualities of the product. But no buyer ever knew for sure if those names really meant anything.

As cannabis has become more widely accepted and used, professional and amateur plant breeders have been developing strains with attributes targeted at specific uses, such as pain relief and help with insomnia. Marketers of these products are finding that customers develop affinities for their favorite strains and tout them on their packaging. These claims seem to be more reliable than those of old-school pot dealers, though they are not tested or regulated by independent agencies.

Strain choices are very prevalent in the marketing of products that contain THC, and they are now becoming more common in CBD products, too. In many cases, the strains have been bred to have very high CBD content or to contain a balance of CBD and THC. (Reminder: Cannabis products containing more than 0.3 percent THC can be sold only in states that permit medical or adult-use marijuana.) But as the CBD market continues to evolve, you can expect that there will be more breeding and marketing of strains for consumers who prefer high CBD cannabis products.

Right now, a few strains are already emerging as popular choices for CBD users. Here are some of the most widely grown.

Charlotte's Web. Probably the best-known strain of high-CBD cannabis, Charlotte's Web was bred by the Stanley brothers in Colorado and was named for a child who suffered from a rare epileptic disorder known as Dravet syndrome, which was relieved by CBD from this strain. The brothers named their CBD brand Charlotte's Web, and they grow and market products made with their proprietary line of this strain. It is very low in THC, so it can be sold nationwide.

Cannatonic was one of the first widely recognized high-CBD strains. It was bred by a CBD genetics company based in Spain called Resin Seeds, which introduced it to the marketplace in 2008. The company reports that half of the plants grown from these seeds will have a 1:1 ratio of CBD to THC. Resin Seeds has since introduced other high-CBD strains such as Dieseltonic and Hammershark.

ACDC (sometimes labeled as "Oracle") is a cross between Cannatonic and *Cannabis ruderalis*, a cannabis species that is naturally low in THC (unlike the more familiar *C. sativa* and *C. indica* types). The ratio of CBD to THC in ACDC is reportedly an average of 20 to 1.

Harlequin comes from several different well-known cannabis strains, such as Thai sativa, Nepalese indica, and a blast from the past, Colombian Gold. Harlequin's 5:2 ratio of CBD to THC has attracted consumers who want the health benefits of CBD along with the psychoactive effects of THC.

Ringo's Gift was named for Lawrence Ringo, a pioneering

advocate for CBD-rich cannabis. It was bred with ACDC, among other strains. While plants grown from Ringo's Gift seeds seem to vary in their CBD to THC ratio, some growers report that it gets to be as high as 24:1.

This information is meant to be helpful for you in choosing cannabis products. But please keep in mind that in many cases products with these strains are still often mislabeled, perhaps inadvertently. More standardization in the CBD industry should lead to more reliability in product labeling.

> **Remember This:** Strains that have high CBD to THC ratios may still contain more than 0.3 percent THC, the legal level for products sold even where medical marijuana is still prohibited.

5 THINGS TO KNOW BEFORE YOU BUY

1. Consider the different delivery systems based on your needs and tastes.
2. Read labels and online product information to learn about a product's origins and manufacturing process.
3. Take note of the type of extract and how it was produced.
4. Look at the certificate of analysis to find out about all of a product's components, including THC level and CBD content.
5. Beware of undesirable additives.

EPILOGUE:
What Comes Next

**THE NEXT FRONTIERS IN HEALTH RESEARCH,
PRODUCTION, AND USAGE.**

The unlikely emergence of CBD as a popular medication would have been hard to predict even just a few years ago. Where it goes from here may be even harder to guess. Some observers from within the CBD world predict that it will someday be as ubiquitous as aspirin, a staple in every home. Others aren't so sure.

"Will it ever be seen as aspirin is? No, I think that is ridiculous," says leading cannabinoid researcher Pal Pacher, M.D., Ph.D., of the NIH. "Aspirin clearly does have some effect on pain, which has been proven in many clinical trials." Dr. Pacher says until CBD's effects are proven in many human studies, he will remain unconvinced. As the past president of the International Cannabis Research Society, he does see potential for cannabidiol as a useful medication for some conditions. He's just not sure what those conditions will be.

"It does not affect one single target in the body. It probably affects 10 or 15 targets. So you cannot link its benefit to one single malady," Dr. Pacher says. "Most likely it is affecting multiple processes and maladies. It makes fully understanding it very difficult. It will take time, but it could be a good thing."

Other experts anticipate that cannabidiol products will settle into a future existence on the shelves of health food stores and vitamin shops. In this scenario, perhaps like a Chinese herbal medicine, CBD will boast a fan base of people who swear by it, while the majority largely ignores it. In fact, at least to one prominent procannabis doctor, the comparison to Chinese medicine is appropriate. Sunil Kumar Aggarwal, M.D., Ph.D., says that, with its popularity, CBD's future is to be the widely accepted substance that will bridge the gap between Western medicine and plant-based healing that's more accepted in Eastern traditions.

Whatever its ultimate fate, the next stage of CBD development will clearly involve lots of study, as researchers try to catch up from the many years lost to the cannabis ban. So many CBD studies are now underway that medical science will certainly be learning much more about the proper dosage, as well as CBD's efficacy for pain, insomnia, anxiety, inflammation, and more. The US Department of Veterans Affairs is already funding its first study of CBD, pairing it with psychotherapy in a treatment for post-traumatic stress disorder (PTSD). The chief investigator says the idea is to break the link between reminders of the trauma and the fear response that it tends to trigger in PTSD sufferers. She says animal models have shown promise and large clinical trials are now underway.

Elsewhere, researchers at New York University are studying CBD as a possible treatment for autism spectrum disorders. In Israel, scientists are investigating whether CBD can calm the immune system enough to help increase the chance of success with bone-marrow transplants. Meanwhile, in Spain, research is underway testing THC and CBD on glioblastoma, the aggressive brain cancer. Other scientists are studying its effect on psychotic disorders, such as schizophrenia. Already, British researchers have noted that giving a single 600 milligram dose of cannabidiol to people suffering with schizophrenia may partially normalize parts of the brain that are known to become dysfunctional during schizophrenic episodes. Some experts see the potential for a medication that may prevent or slow the disease.

As more studies are completed and years go by, researchers will also learn much more about the long-term effects of cannabidiol. Israeli research presented at the American Epilepsy Society's annual meeting in 2018 indicated that perhaps CBD's benefits may start to fade for some patients after about seven months of use, requiring a dosage increase for about a third of patients. More study will yield more specific recommendations. It's also likely that the endocannabinoid system will be taught more widely in medical schools, leading to increased understanding by the professional medical community.

One consequence of the Farm Bill is that more cannabidiol will be harvested from US farms, as many regions in the United States are suitable for growing hemp. In the past, companies often imported hemp from countries such as Romania, Hungary, Russia, Canada, and, the biggest producer, China. This change may affect the products consumers can buy. Some observers predict that the domestic hemp supply may be less contaminated by pesticides than some imported hemp. And since costs to obtain the hemp could fall, companies may eventually lower consumer prices.

At the same time, the market is expected to grow exponentially. Most observers of the CBD industry, whether they are proponents or skeptics, see the boom continuing in coming years. *Forbes* estimates that there are as many as 1,000 CBD-infused products available online already with many more coming. The market research firm Brightfield Group has predicted that between 2018 and 2023 the year-over-year growth rate will reach 107 percent. In other words, the industry will more than double in sales every year.

Analysts say that a big part of the growth will come from areas such as cosmetics and food and drink products. Already, many CBD lotions and balms are available from new companies as well as venerable brands, such as Estée Lauder, which has introduced a hydrating face mask infused with cannabidiol. Many companies are awaiting FDA approval allowing them to add cannabidiol into a wide range of grocery products, including soda, beer, and water.

Some experts worry that the hype around CBD has set up false expectations that it will never live up to. Others are concerned that, with all the money already involved, the merchandising will outweigh the medical benefits and CBD will eventually be seen mainly as a marketable commodity, found on store shelves but not taken seriously as a useful medication.

In the end, knowing exactly what CBD will become is impossible. A niche supplement for natural-healing advocates who appreciate their medications in a plant-based package? A gimmicky ingredient adding a vague sense of wellness to everyday products? A critical answer for certain types of epilepsy and other major diseases? A mainstream solution found in most medicine cabinets to treat pain, inflammation, sleeplessness, and anxiety? Or something else we can't yet imagine? Linked to one of the body's most important systems and to one of the planet's most controversial plants, its history kept cannabidiol cloaked in mystery until recently. One thing is certain. It is hidden no longer. For some, CBD remains all hype. For others, it represents hope. And ultimately, when telling the tale of CBD, this is the critical judgment. Hype or hope? In time, we all may find out. But for now, you get to decide.

Resources

WHERE TO GO FOR MORE INFORMATION

NONPROFITS AND TRADE GROUPS

Hemp Industries Association
https://www.thehia.org

National Cannabis Industry Association
https://thecannabisindustry.org

National Hemp Association
https://nationalhempassociation.org

Project CBD
https://www.projectcbd.org

U.S. Hemp Authority
ushempauthority.org

INSTITUTIONAL RESEARCH

Center for Medical Cannabis Research,
University of California at San Diego
https://www.cmcr.ucsd.edu

International Cannabinoid Research Society
https://icrs.co/

International Research Center on Cannabis and Health
https://ircch.com

National Institutes of Health Research on
Marijuana and Cannabinoids
https://www.drugabuse.gov/drugs-abuse/marijuana/
nih-research-marijuana-cannabinoids

STUDIES CITED IN THIS BOOK
(IN ORDER OF CITATION IN THE BOOK)

The health effects of cannabis and cannabinoids:
the current state of evidence and recommendations
National Academy of Sciences
https://www.nap.edu/catalog/24625/the-health-effects-of-
cannabis-and-cannabinoids-the-current-state

Cannabidiol (CBD) Critical Review Report
World Health Organization: Expert Committee on Drug
Dependency, Fortieth Meeting, Geneva, June 4-7, 2018
https://www.who.int/medicines/access/controlled-substances/
CannabidiolCriticalReview.pdf

Cannabinoids in attention-deficit/hyperactivity disorder:
A randomised-controlled trial
Journal of the European College of Neuropsychopharmacology,
May 2017
https://www.ncbi.nlm.nih.gov/pubmed/28576350

Early phase in the development of cannabidiol as a treatment
for addiction: opioid relapse takes initial center stage
Neurotherapeutics, August 2015
https://www.ncbi.nlm.nih.gov/pmc/articles/PMC4604178/

Cannabidiol reduces cigarette consumption in tobacco smokers: preliminary findings
Addictive Behaviors, April 2013
https://www.ncbi.nlm.nih.gov/pubmed/23685330

Neural basis of anxiolytic effects of cannabidiol (CBD) in generalized social anxiety disorder: a preliminary report
Journal of Psychopharmacology, September 2010
https://journals.sagepub.com/doi/abs/10.1177/0269881110379283

Cannabidiol as a potential treatment for anxiety disorders
Neurotherapeutics, September 2015
https://www.ncbi.nlm.nih.gov/pmc/articles/PMC4604171/

Cannabidiol as a therapeutic alternative for post-traumatic stress disorder: from bench research to confirmation in human trials
Frontiers in Neuroscience, July 2018
https://www.frontiersin.org/articles/10.3389/fnins.2018.00502/full

Transdermal cannabidiol reduces inflammation and pain-related behaviours in a rat model of arthritis
European Journal of Pain, July 2016
https://www.ncbi.nlm.nih.gov/pmc/articles/PMC4851925/

Cannabidiol to Improve Mobility in People with Multiple Sclerosis
Frontiers in Neurology, March 2018
https://www.frontiersin.org/articles/10.3389/fneur.2018.00183/full

The non-psychoactive cannabis constituent cannabidiol is an orally effective therapeutic agent in rat chronic inflammatory and neuropathic pain.
European Journal of Pharmacology, February 2007
https://www.ncbi.nlm.nih.gov/pubmed/17157290

Cannabidiol lowers incidence of diabetes in non-obese diabetic mice
Autoimmunity, March 2006
https://www.ncbi.nlm.nih.gov/pubmed/16698671

Cannabis use in patients with fibromyalgia:
effect on symptoms relief and health-related quality of life
Public Library of Science (PLOS) One, April 2011
https://www.ncbi.nlm.nih.gov/pubmed/21533029

A single dose of cannabidiol reduces blood pressure in healthy volunteers in a randomized crossover study
Journal of Clinical Insight, June 2017
https://insight.jci.org/articles/view/93760

The endocannabinoid system in guarding against fear, anxiety and stress
Nature Review Neuroscience, November 2015
https://www.nature.com/articles/nrn4036

Cannabidiol in anxiety and sleep: a large case series
Permanente Journal, January 2019
https://www.ncbi.nlm.nih.gov/pmc/articles/PMC6326553/

Regulation of nausea and vomiting by cannabinoids
British Journal of Pharmacology, August 2011
https://www.ncbi.nlm.nih.gov/pubmed/21175589

Cannabinoid receptors and the regulation of bone mass
British Journal of Pharmacology, January 2008
https://www.ncbi.nlm.nih.gov/pmc/articles/PMC2219540/

Cannabidiol for the treatment of psychosis in Parkinson's disease
Journal of Psychopharmacology, September 2008
https://journals.sagepub.com/doi/
abs/10.1177/0269881108096519

Cannabidiol can improve complex sleep-related behaviours
associated with rapid eye movement sleep behaviour disorder
in Parkinson's disease patients: a case series
Journal of Clinical Pharmacy and Therapeutics, May 2014
https://onlinelibrary.wiley.com/doi/abs/10.1111/jcpt.12179

Cannabidiol treatment for refractory seizures in
sturge-weber syndrome
Pediatric Neurology, June 2017
https://www.sciencedirect.com/science/article/abs/pii/
S088789941730053X

The role of cannabinoids in dermatology
Journal of the American Academy of Dermatology, July 2017
https://www.jaad.org/article/S0190-9622(17)30308-0/abstract

Labeling accuracy of cannabidiol extracts sold online
Journal of the American Medical Association, November 2017
https://jamanetwork.com/journals/jama/fullarticle/2661569

Index

CBD *(continued)*

how it works, 17
isolates, 69, 71, 75, 123, 140–41, 153
legal status of, 18–19, 56–58, 141
manufacture of, 65–66
market growth and, 14–15, 162–63
most popular uses for, 12, 17–18, 21–27
myths about, 72–83
for pets *(see* pets, CBD for)
popularity of, 13–14, 15, 50–51
potential uses for, 20, 89–90, 160–61
    (see also specific conditions)
quality control and, 36–38, 134–35
    (see also quality issues)
resources on, 165–69
safety of, 19, 31, 76–79
strains of, 155–57
terpenes and, 67–68, 69, 70, 81
vs. THC, 48, 62
user experiences with, 14, 15, 18, 30,
    36, 44, 51, 52, 57, 72, 105, 130, 154
World Health Organization on, 88
CBD products. *See also* CBD
availability of, 119–20
FDA restrictions on, 87–88, 127, 132
ingestible, 16
    capsules and softgels, 67, 122–23,
        145, 151, 153
    CBD-enhanced foods, 127–28, 145,
        162, 163
    dab, wax, and shatter, 129–30,
        136–37
    edibles, 125–26, 142
    fizzy tablets, 123
    functional foods, 126, 145
    oral or nasal sprays, 125, 153
    sublingual strips, 124–25
    tinctures, 43, 66, 123–24, 142–43,
        145, 153, 154
    vape oil, 67, 128–29, 136, 143–44,
        151, 153
mislabeling of, 74, 78, 121–22, 134–35,
    157
misleading claims about, 79–80, 81–83
with THC added, 141–42
THC content in, 38, 56, 57, 58, 69–70,
    71, 73, 74–75, 118, 135, 141

topical, 16, 130
    bath bombs and salts, 132–33
    cosmetics, 79–80, 131–32, 151, 162,
        163
    lotions, creams, and balms, 66, 131,
        144, 153, 162–63
    skin patches, 133
    traveling with, 75
CB1 receptors, 63, 65
CB2 receptors, 63, 65, 68, 106
certificate of analysis (COA), 38, 147, 148,
    152, 153, 157
Charlotte's Web strain, 153, 156
chemical sensitivity, 154
chemotherapy, 21, 87, 104
China
    early cannabis use in, 40, 85
    hemp grown in, 62
chronic pain, 87, 132
    CBD for, 24, 57, 96–97, 105, 131, 150
    medical marijuana for, 24–25
    in pets, 113
clobazam, CBD interaction with, 76
Comprehensive Drug Abuse Prevention
        and Control Act, 46–47
concentrates, 129–30, 136–37
cosmetics, 131–32, 151, 162, 163
creams, 131, 153
CV Sciences, 153
CW Hemp, 153

D

dab, 129–30, 136–37
decarboxylation, 137, 138–39
Depakene, CBD interaction with, 76
diabetes, 97–98
DIY extraction methods, 137–38
dosage recommendations, 34–36, 88–89,
    144
    for pets, 115–16
Dravet syndrome, 27, 87, 108, 109, 156
drug interactions, CBD and, 76–77, 88,
    117
drug tests, 73–75

E

eating disorders, 99–100
edibles, 125–26, 142. *See also* gummies
Egypt, early cannabis use in, 40
endocannabinoid system (ECS), 17, 49, 50, 62–65, 68, 96, 100, 102–3, 106, 110, 111, 113, 161–62
England, early hemp use in, 41
entourage effect, 69–71, 140, 142
Epidiolex, for epilepsy, 27–28, 29, 32, 49, 77, 87, 110
epilepsy, 27–29, 30, 49, 55, 56, 82–83, 87, 89, 108–11, 144, 156. *See also* seizures
    in pets, 114, 115
extraction methods, 61, 121, 135–39

F

Farm Bill, 18, 47, 50, 57, 162
fibromyalgia, 100–101, 133, 154
fizzy tablets, 123
Food and Drug Administration (FDA)
    CBD restrictions and, 87–88, 127, 132
    Epidiolex approved by, 27, 29, 30, 32, 49, 87
    labeling regulations of, 144, 146–47
foods, CBD-enhanced, 126–28, 145, 162, 163
foot pain, 132
full-spectrum CBD, 69–70, 71, 74, 122, 139–40, 141
functional foods, 126, 145

G

ginger, 86
gummies, 66–67, 125, 145, 153
Gupta, Sanjay, 55–56

H

Harlequin strain, 156
headaches, 18
hemp
    components of, 69, 139–40
    defined, 141
    growing, 61–62, 65, 149–50
    history of, 39–40, 41–43
    imported, 162
    industrial uses for, 41, 42, 61
    legalization of, 18, 47, 50, 57, 58
    organic, 118, 148
    origin of, 145–46
    terpenes in, 67, 68
    THC content in, 13, 57, 62
    versatile uses for, 120
hemp extract, 122, 145, 151, 153
hemp seed oil, 120–21
heroin addiction, 83, 92
hot flashes, 102, 105
hydrocarbon extraction, 136–37

I

India, early cannabis use in, 40, 85
inflammation
    arthritis and, 94, 95
    autoimmune disorders and, 95, 96
    CBD relieving, 17, 18, 21, 22, 24, 25–26
ingestible CBD products. *See* CBD products, ingestible
insomnia, 11, 12, 14, 18, 22, 52, 92, 101–2
isolates, 69, 71, 75, 123, 140–41, 153

J

Jefferson, Thomas, 42

L

label language, 144–46
laboratory testing, 146–48
Lazarus Naturals, 153
Lennox-Gastaut syndrome, 27, 87, 108, 109
linalool, 68
liver, effect of CBD on, 76, 77–78, 88
Loewe, Walter S., 48
lotions, 131, 144, 162–63

M

Marihuana Tax Act, 46
marijuana
    ancient writings on, 40

marijuana *(continued)*

Notes